What's your NUMBER?
the palmer code

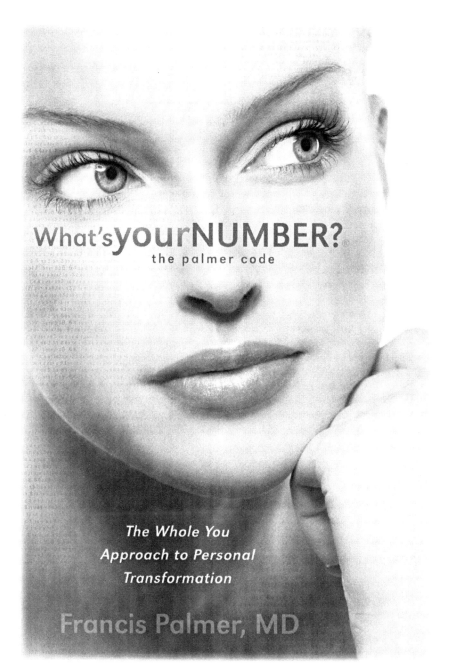

What's your NUMBER?
the palmer code

The Whole You Approach to Personal Transformation

Francis Palmer, MD

New York

What's Your Number?
The Palmer Code
The Whole You Approach to Personal Transformation

Copyright 2009 Francis Palmer, MD. All rights reserved.

No part of this publication may be reproduced or transmitted in any form or by any means, mechanical or electronic, including photocopying and recording, or by any information storage and retrieval system, without permission in writing from the author or publisher (except by a reviewer, who may quote brief passages and/or short brief video clips in a review.)

Disclaimer: The Publisher and the Author make no representations or warranties with respect to the accuracy or completeness of the contents of this work and specifically disclaim all warranties, including without limitation warranties of fitness for a particular purpose. No warranty may be created or extended by sales or promotional materials. The advice and strategies contained herein may not be suitable for every situation. This work is sold with the understanding that the Publisher is not engaged in rendering legal, accounting, or other professional services. If professional assistance is required, the services of a competent professional person should be sought. Neither the Publisher nor the Author shall be liable for damages arising herefrom. The fact that an organization or website is referred to in this work as a citation and/or a potential source of further information does not mean that the Author or the Publisher endorses the information the organization or website may provide or recommendations it may make. Further, readers should be aware that internet websites listed in this work may have changed or disappeared between when this work was written and when it is read.

Softcover ISBN 978-1-60037-580-4
Hardcover ISBN 978-1-60037-581-1

MORGAN · JAMES
THE ENTREPRENEURIAL PUBLISHER

Morgan James Publishing, LLC
1225 Franklin Ave., STE 325
Garden City, NY 11530-1693
Toll Free 800-485-4943
www.MorganJamesPublishing.com

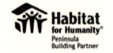

In an effort to support local communities, raise awareness and funds, Morgan James Publishing donates one percent of all book sales for the life of each book to Habitat for Humanity. Get involved today, visit www.HelpHabitatForHumanity.org.

Table of Contents

Preface: The Self-Realization Theory of Everything *1*
What is the Palmer Code? 3
The Principles of the Palmer Code 3

Chapter 1: The Emotion of Beauty *7*
The Palmer Code 8
Self-Esteem 10
Why I'm Writing This Book 11

Chapter 2: Why Know Your Number *15*
The Palmer Code Principles 15
What Your Number Can Do for You 19
The Number of the Common Man 20

Chapter 3: The Palmer Code and Your Number *23*
Beauty Equations 24
The Whole Number Components 25
A Closer Look at the Outer you 27
Facial Components 27
The Body 30
Skin (overall) 31
Hair 31
Grooming 31
Style 32
The Inner You 32
Bringing it all Together 34

Chapter 4: The Palmer Code for the Face 35

Facial Shapes 35
Face Shapes on Profile 36
The Sexes 37
Facial Features 37
The Big Three 37
Calculating your Cheek Volume 38
The Eyes and Eyebrows 40
The Lips 40
The Nose 41
The Rest 43
The Neck 43
The Jaw 43
The Chin 44
The Skin 44
How It All Comes Together 45

Chapter 5: Your Own Face Number and the Big Three 47

How to Calculate Your Own Face Number 48
The Cheeks 48
Female Cheeks 49
Male Cheeks 50
Eyes and Eyebrows (Eye Area) 51
Female Eye Area: 51
Male Eye Area: 52
Lips 52

Chapter 6: Your Own Face Number for the Rest 55

Skin 55
Jaw Line, Neck, and Chin 56
Nose 57
Overall Flow 58

Chapter 7: Unlocking Your Face's Beauty Potential 63

Exercise One 63
Exercise Two 65
Exercise Three 66
Baseline 68
Makeup by the Numbers 68
Cheeks 69
Eyes and Eyebrows 70
Lips 72
The Nose and the Rest of Your Face 74
Your Hair 76

vi

Exercise is an Important Key to Your Face Number 77
Cheek muscles 77
Eye Area (Eye and Eyebrow) Muscles 78
Toning the neck 79
Skin Care and the Palmer Code 80
Skin Care Steps 82
Weight Gain and Loss to Shape the face 84
Beautiful Teeth Enhance Your Smile 84
A Full, Thick Head of Hair 85

Chapter 8: The Palmer Code Body *87*
Body Evaluation 89
Upper-to-Lower Body Ratio 89
Hips 92
Legs (Men) 93
Chest 94
Buttocks 95
Abdomen 96
Shoulders and Arms 97
Skin 98
Your Body Prescription 99

Chapter 9: Women, Unlock Your Palmer Code Body *101*
Upper-to-Lower Body Ratio 101
Hips and Legs 102
Breasts 103
Buttocks 104
Abdomen 105
Shoulders and Arms 106
Skin 106
The Female Form 106

Chapter 10: Men, Unlock Your Palmer Code Body *109*
Upper-to-lower body ratio 109
Hips and Waist 110
Legs 111
Chest 111
Buttocks 112
Abdomen 112
Shoulders 113
Arms 114
Skin 114
The Male Physique 115

vii

Chapter 11: Supporting Factors *117*
   Skin. 117
   Hair. 119
   Other Outer You Components 120
   Style. 122
   The Outer you. 122

Chapter 12: The Inner You *123*
   The Mysteries of Attraction 123
   Components of the Inner You 125
   Physical Well-Being and the Palmer Code 128
   Shining Your Light. 128

Chapter 13: Unlocking the Inner You *131*
   Physical Well-Being Analysis 132
   Emotional Well-Being Analysis 133
   Understanding Your Inner You Number 134
   Stress 138
   Habits 142

Chapter 14: Achieve and Maintain Your Number and Best Self *143*
   Maintaining Your Number for the Face 143
   Maintaining Your Number for the Body 144
   Maintaining Your Skin (Same Principles As The Face) 145
   Maintaining Your Hair. 145
   Maintaining Your Emotional Health and Your Number within the
      Inner You 145
   Maintaining Your Physical Health and Your Number within the
      Inner You 146
   Establishing the Habit 147
   Your Palmer Code Self. 151

Chapter 15: Afterword *153*

Appendix A: What's Your Number® Worksheet. *157*
   What's Your Number®?. 157

Appendix B: Ideal Weight Charts. *163*

About the Author. *167*

Book Bonus *169*

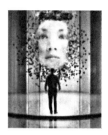

Preface: The Self-Realization Theory of Everything

Self-realization is defined as the development or fulfillment of one's full potential. Consider that for a moment. Is there some aspect of your life that is yet to be fulfilled?

The *Palmer Code* reveals how completely our appearance is integrated, intertwined, and affected by every aspect of our lives. It's all the things that make us who and what we are: how we feel, our overall physical health, relationships, sense of self-worth, emotional state, education, living conditions, physical features, sense of style, stress at home or at work along with any and everything else that make us unique as individuals. These things are all directly related to, affected by, and dependent upon one another to such an extent that they simply can't be separated.

Think about it. If you are self-confident, doesn't this affect how you feel and doesn't the way that you feel have an impact on how you look? This in turn affects how you deal with your relationships, that impacts your emotional state, decreases your stress levels and provides positive factors in your overall health… and on and on it goes. This simple, yet effective thought exercise demonstrates just the tip of the iceberg, because the secrets of the *Palmer Code* are far more encompassing. That's why understanding this revolutionary concept and learning how to incorporate its fundamental principles and secrets will empower you to make life-altering changes.

Early on, when I was developing the inner workings of the *Palmer Code*, something remarkable happened. As I sat contemplating the impact of the various *Code* elements, a singular moment of clarity revealed to me the complexity, intertwined nature, and complete integration of our appearance with every aspect of daily life. I remember the incredible impact of that moment. Like an ever expanding ripple, created from dropping a stone into a still pond, my mind began racing in all directions as I thought of more and more facets of our humanity that appeared to be inescapably connected to our outward appearance.

At first, I resisted the sheer scope of it and thought "surely this can't be correct." In those first few moments, as I struggled to come to grips with this marvelous revelation, I tried to imagine anything that could not be addressed by the principles behind the *Palmer Code*. However, try as I might, I couldn't come up with a single facet of human life that didn't somehow interact with and affect how we look, and vice versa. I then remembered, other ideas that found simplicity in the seemingly complex, like the concept of "six degrees of separation" that states we are all somehow related to every other person on this planet within a maximum of six relationships or Einstein's equation $E = MC^2$.

I came to realize that beauty really is related to all the various and diverse aspects of our human existence. A simple truth defining a seemingly complex and random part of nature—beauty and our everyday lives. I recall having chills at that very moment when the true power and simple truth contained within the *Palmer Code* was revealed. It was, for me, a profound moment of inspiration, enlightenment and encouragement. Simple, yet infinitely powerful, it is the "theory of everything" as it relates to how we live, feel and look as human beings. I vowed there and then to share this good news with the rest of the world.

The *Palmer Code* will help you make dramatic, sometimes life-altering changes by understanding the relationships that all the seemingly disconnected parts of your daily activities have with your appearance. You'll learn the secrets of how to improve your mind, body, attitude, physical appearance and so much more by making simple, yet profound changes in the way you do the things you already do. Use the *Palmer Code* as your ultimate self-help, self-realization and self-improvement guide. The secrets are all here for you to make the *best possible you* inside and out.

What is the Palmer Code?

When you look in the mirror, what do you see? Do you ever wonder if you see yourself the same way others see you? Do you feel like you have control of improving your appearance and your life?

Most of us take care of ourselves and our looks, investing in shampoos, make-up, clothing, exercise and healthy eating because we believe these will help us to look and feel our best. The question is, do we really understand all the possible contributing factors and are we investing our time and money in a way that will pay off by creating real and substantial improvement? What if there was a scientific approach to make sure that when you step out into the world, you always look and feel your absolute best? Now imagine, what if you could apply that same scientific approach to all aspects of your life? That's the promise of the *Palmer Code*.

The Principles of the Palmer Code

After nearly two decades of medical practice, research and analysis, I have unlocked the secrets of what makes us beautiful, and identified the tremendous impact that the various factors of our daily lives have on our appearance. The *Palmer Code* unlocks real solutions for optimal living through scientific algorithms that define beauty's component parts. It exposes the undeniable association of our appearance with all facets of life and then provides simple solutions for total self improvement, both inside and out.

The Palmer Code is the first book in a series devoted to optimum living. It outlines the way to self-improvement in a three-step approach that balances *information* with *analysis* in order to create *successful change*. In other words, you *learn first, analyze second* and then you *take action*. Sound simple? It is. And yet we tend to get lost in the

The Palmer Code [Francis Palmer MD]

chaos of information bombarding us from the fashion, health and cosmetics industries. If you're looking to improve your appearance, does it really make sense to aim for sunken cheeks and blackout eye shadow on a super-skinny body? As a plastic and cosmetic surgeon in Beverly Hills where celebrities set the standard for world class beauty, I have determined the core elements that comprise *ideal beauty* and the many ways you can approach that ideal. Sometimes the answer can be as simple as changing your hair, make-up, attitude, eating habits and clothing. The *Palmer Code* philosophy applies to all walks of life and utilizes simple logical steps towards optimal living.

The *Palmer Code* principles involve three simple steps:

1. Define the key elements
2. Evaluate yourself
3. Focus on what's important, and don't worry about the rest

The secret to this approach is in the balance. For example, by knowing that the *inner you* accounts for 40% of how you appear to the world, it becomes apparent that your feelings and emotions have a direct and powerful impact on how good you look. You can take your image to the next level through adjustments in your mood and your attitude towards yourself and others, as well as lifestyle changes like eliminating stress, healthy eating and regular exercise.

As you delve further into the *Palmer Code* and how to analyze the *outer you*—your physical appearance—you'll learn among other things that the eye area (eyes/eyebrows), incorrectly touted as the most important beauty feature of the face, actually account for only 10% of what makes the face beautiful. Even more surprising to some, the nose and skin contribute even less. After learning these facts, you may be more likely to reach for a pair of tweezers than worry about that smattering of freckles across your nose. As a society, we waste a lot of time and money trying to fix things that just aren't important. That's because we simply were never taught what counts when it comes to ideal beauty. Until now. Using the *Palmer Code* to determine which aspects of your appearance hold priority, you can set a beauty baseline. From there, you determine which areas to improve, which ones are already great and which ones to forget about.

The *Palmer Code* guides you through the many ways that you can make changes in your daily activities, creating dramatic improvements not only in your appearance but in your entire life. Imagine the power you'll have over your life when you consider how all things are interconnected and most importantly, truly under your control. Physical health, exercise program, relationships, eating habits, hair style, clothing, self-esteem, career, living conditions, work environment, attitude, emotions, mental health and physical features—you'll understand how to optimize everything. Best of all, when you improve one aspect of your life, it has a ripple effect upon all aspects of your life. What could be more powerful? Using the *Palmer Code*, you are the master of your own destiny. In complete control over the creation of the best you that you can possibly be. The *Palmer Code* is the self realization theory of everything.

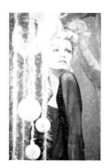

Chapter 1: The Emotion of Beauty

Make-up accentuates her eyes in dark, dramatic colors. Her nails are painted orange. She wears gold and silver necklaces and bracelets studded with jewels. On her head are: hair extensions tamed with pomade. Who is she? Quite simply, a woman. One who lived four thousand years ago in ancient Egypt.

Funny, but we tend to think of beauty obsession as a modern-day phenomenon. Not true. In ancient Egypt there was no stigma associated with vanity. They celebrated their appearance for social and sexual reasons, but they also believed their looks held a direct relationship to the spirit. They made their eye make-up out of kohl, nail polish from henna and blush from red clay. Surprisingly, it wasn't just women, either; men used various fats to combat balding. The ancient Egyptians believed in regular bathing, keeping a neat appearance and smelling nice. We only know about this because they also happened to keep really good records. It's possible that grooming and beauty practices dated back even further than that. Who knows?

Nowadays, though, there does seem to be a trend in mass self-consciousness. Go anywhere in public—even if you just throw on your sweats to grab some coffee—and you could wind up in a photograph or even on video. Cameras are everywhere, even on our cell phones and digital photographs can have a shelf life of... well, for as long as the Internet exists. We all have a vague sense of what makes us look good. But do we really know how to look our absolute best?

The Palmer Code   [Francis Palmer MD]

My name is Dr. Francis Palmer and I'm a Beverly Hills plastic and cosmetic surgeon. I make people more attractive for a living. That's my job and for over 18 years, on two continents, I have evaluated and improved the appearance of thousands and thousands of people. From heads of state, royalty and celebrities, to the average guy, I have been called upon to do just one simple thing: Make these people more attractive. I've done this in a precise and predictable manner using the *Palmer Code*, but things weren't always so obvious in the early days as I was starting out. I trained for 10 years to learn my craft in plastic and cosmetic surgery, yet as I began my practice, there was a nagging sense that something was missing. Some vital key element that if found, would complete my knowledge and training. I didn't realize it then, but that something was a clear definition of human beauty.

Several years later, after much study and observation, I realized there was a pattern to what we, as a society, deem attractive. Some things were obvious of course, but others, not so much. I wondered if it was possible to demystify beauty. I began searching until I was able to formulate that definition into a repeatable, predictable algorithm. Since then, I've used this algorithm countless times to make my patients more attractive. To me, that's the ultimate proof of concept.

Over the years, I came to realize that there are many components from the obvious hair style and makeup, to the seemingly obscure factors of daily life like emotion and physical health that affect and are affected by our appearance. Can these factors be incorporated into the beauty algorithm? Turns out they can. The *Palmer Code* was born.

The Palmer Code

Put a hundred people in a room. Ask them if they think Angelina Jolie, Catherine Zeta Jones, Brad Pitt, Marilyn Monroe and George Clooney are beautiful. Most people will agree that yes, they're gorgeous people but if you ask them to define what makes some people beautiful and others not, you'll get 100 different answers. Beauty has always been tough to define. People consider it subjective and even harder to quantify.

8

[Francis Palmer MD] The Palmer Code

After nearly two decades of plastic and cosmetic surgery practice, I discovered that it's possible to express not only the way you look but the *whole you* with a single number between 1 and 100. I call it the *Palmer Code*. Once you know the secrets, contained within my *beauty code*, you can not only determine *your number*, you can use simple tricks of hair style, make-up, exercise, healthy living, attitude adjustment, improving relationships, building self-esteem, finding tranquility in life and work to maximize

> • • •
>
> **"It's possible to express the way you look with a single number."**
>
> • • •

not only your beauty, but your entire life. You can achieve full self-realization and unlock your full life potential.

The *Palmer Code* takes into account both your physical beauty and your inner self, and translates it into a single, all-encompassing number. This number (*your number*) personifies the *whole you* or your *whole self*, which is the way you're seen by society and the people around you. Many factors influence *your number*, some for better, some for worse but by determining *your number* and establishing a baseline, you reveal the countless ways you can work to improve your appearance and your life.

People evaluate one another every day. They compare one person to the next, assess levels of attraction and categorize. It happens so fast and at such a subconscious level that most people are unaware they're even doing it, but they are. In a way, a first impression is an instant assessment of *your number*. When you wake up and brush your teeth, style your hair, select a nice outfit, hit the gym, or pursue any other healthy habit, you're making conscious decisions that affect *your number*.

The *Palmer Code* offers a clear way for people to look at themselves. It's like a life improvement roadmap. You use it every day—whether you're washing your face, going to yoga class, meditating or putting on lipstick—as a way to make better decisions about yourself and your appearance. Beauty is just a part of *your number* within the *Palmer*

The Palmer Code [Francis Palmer MD]

Code, but beauty is also extremely powerful in modern society. In our youth and beauty-oriented culture, there's no question that some of the world's most adored and successful celebrities are beautiful. Case in point, using the *Palmer Code*, Angelina Jolie's *face number* is a perfect 100 and Jennifer Aniston's is a 99. Both women are gorgeous because they exhibit many of the ideal beauty characteristics found within the *Palmer Code*. In fact, it turns out that many celebrities have higher *numbers* than the average person. Could this be part of the reason that they are constantly sought by their adoring fans? It sure doesn't hurt and if it helps celebrities gain power, wealth and fame, what if you could use it to your advantage as well? Isn't it only natural for us to be curious and ask, *"what's my number?"* After reading *The Palmer Code*, I'm certain that you'll not only want to know *your number*, you'll know what you'd like that number to become. Beauty often serves as its own motivation. As Truman Capote said, "beauty makes its own rules."

Self-Esteem

Fortunately, in today's society, there seems to be less of a stigma associated with wanting to improve your looks. I've come to understand how appearance can boost someone's confidence. An extreme example of this occurred a few years ago, when I donated plastic surgery services on a pro bono case. The patient, a victim of domestic violence, had been beaten so badly that her face was left scarred and disfigured. She felt self-conscious and reclusive, afraid to socialize or seek employment.

> • • •
> **"Transform into your physical ideal."**
> • • •

I performed surgery, repaired the damage and restored the essential beauty in her face using the principles of my *beauty code*. Afterward, she said she felt empowered. She got a new job, became more involved in her children's activities and moved forward with her life. Could she have done these things without having her appearance altered? Of course, and yet the power of self-confidence is undeniable.

Why I'm Writing This Book

Most of us will never have to know what it's like to live with a physical disfigurement. However, we do know the power that comes from looking and feeling our best. By applying the science of the *Palmer Code* to make simple changes in your appearance and the various facets of your everyday life, you undergo a metamorphosis. You transform into your physical and mental ideal.

From the beginning as a plastic and cosmetic surgeon, I never believed beauty was esoteric. If that were true, then why is there collective agreement on what constitutes what I call *"star-quality gorgeous"* and even more importantly how could I consistently make people more attractive in the OR? In my career, I've studied many beautiful faces and I have indeed recognized recurring patterns not only in beauty but in people's behavior and reaction to the way they look.

Unfortunately, people don't always make the right choices when dealing with their appearance and over the years I've seen many who've made poor decisions about cosmetic surgery. Some I've been able to help, while others were not so fortunate. I understand how something like that could happen because my knowledge of beauty came from self-study and insight, not from conventional training. It may surprise you to learn that plastic and cosmetic surgeons are taught to perform surgical procedures. They're not necessarily taught to understand, define and recognize what beauty is, which makes it much more difficult to create.

In fact, few people truly understand beauty. It's as if you need to look at it through an artist's eyes. I often find that I have to teach my patients what will and what won't make them more attractive. I've even had to get tough with patients who approach cosmetic surgery too lightly. For instance, I find many people are way too casual about rhinoplasty (nose jobs). Contrary to popular belief, you can't keep hopping from surgeon to surgeon, asking them to operate on your nose until it's perfect. It's an invasive procedure! I'm not saying there aren't times when rhinoplasty is appropriate, but the truth is, the nose carries much less aesthetic importance than generally believed. It's also true

The Palmer Code [Francis Palmer MD]

that in some cases, simple make-up tricks can be used to make the nose blend into the face, allowing the "best" aesthetic features to emerge.

The Palmer Code not only defines what beauty is, but what it is not, by debunking disturbing trends like the extremely thin, unhealthy role models so prevalent in Hollywood today. They may be thin, but they are not attractive. Since when did skin and bones become beautiful?

Another important factor in assessing *your number* is the *inner you*—your inner beauty, an area frequently overlooked and under-estimated. However, since modern society places such a premium on youth and beauty, you would be foolish to overlook any advantage because the simple fact is real beauty equates to power. If a real beauty enters a room, heads will turn.

I realize that this concept will seem controversial to some. It might appear that I am boiling everything in life down to the essence of a single number at the expense of humanity. Nothing could be farther from the truth. I believe that beauty, in the human form, can be ascertained. If you want to become more attractive there are ways to make that happen. I'm writing this book to give you the inside scoop on how you can get an edge and how you can make the most of *your number*. That is my intent.

You may not realize it, but your *Palmer Code number* is already part of your daily routine. Do you shower, shampoo your hair, and brush your teeth in the morning? Do you consider what clothes you wear? Do you take time to do your hair and put on makeup? Do you exercise? Do you try to maintain a healthy body and mind? If so, why? These are all ways to enhance or maintain *your number*.

By now, I hope it's obvious that the *Palmer Code* isn't just for people caught up in the latest fad or trends in health, diets, beauty products and cosmetic surgery. It's for anyone interested in looking and feeling his or her best. By understanding the various factors within *your number*, you can make your everyday routines even more effective. You can feel great and look even better.

I believe that people are genetically programmed to respond to beauty and beautiful people. I believe that it's not only quite natural to crave real beauty, it's part of human nature to strive for its achievement in all things. Is it wrong to strive for beauty? I don't think so.

Me, I love to paint landscape and seascape scenes. The process itself is relaxing and it feels good to create something beautiful. I feel a sense of delight while I'm painting and I enjoy the finished work when it hangs in my home or office. Many have experienced the joy of beauty, for beauty's sake. They say that Buddha himself once conducted an entire sermon without speaking a single word. He simply held up a lotus flower and gazed upon it. I can't speak on the principles of Buddhism, but whether you're Buddhist or Hindu or Christian as I am, I do believe it's a gift—not a burden—that we, as humans, can enjoy and appreciate real beauty in all things, including ourselves.

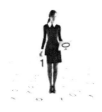

Chapter 2:
Why Know Your Number

The Palmer Code Principles

To understand why you should know *your number*, you first need to understand what a *Palmer Code number* is. *Your number* is simply a code based on each piece that makes up the *outer you* and the *inner you*. Think of it as a blending of science and beauty.

All things have an aesthetic profile, from people or flowers to the chair, bed, or sofa you might be sitting on right now. The study of aesthetic science has existed throughout history and it's been measured by the greatest philosophers, scientists and mathematicians of all time. Think Leonardo Da Vinci, who obsessively combined beauty with invention; or Pythagoras, whose golden ratio (figure 2-2) has defined aesthetic ideals in art, architecture and even music. What's amazing about the golden ratio (characterized by the Greek letter phi Φ) is that it acts as a pivotal key that unlocks both art and mathematics and depending on who you're talking to, many other sciences and beliefs.

Using my *Code*, you calculate each component of *your number* by using three golden steps:

1. Define key elements
2. Evaluate
3. Focus on improving what's important

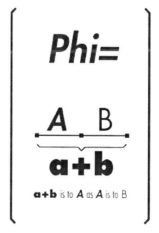

Figure 2-2

The Palmer Code [Francis Palmer MD]

Let's take a look at how this works using something familiar to many of you: home improvement, or more specifically, *garden* improvement, as an example.

Define key elements

Picture yourself in a woodland garden. Fallen leaves and sticks are tangled in with violets, lilies, roses climbing on an arbor, and some hostas and ferns in the shadier spots beneath trees that are filled with birds. The flowers are beautiful and fragrant, but they're jumbled around one another and a few weeds have taken root. There's also a cracked birdbath in the center of the garden, and a sparkling jasmine-rimmed stream that winds around the perimeter.

With one look, your brain registers that this is a nice garden that is imperfect. You also realize that with a little care, it could be spectacular. But how do you get it that way?

To begin, you take a look at the key elements. In any garden, aesthetic design begins with structure. The flowers are nice but they're so tangled together that as a component, they become weaker. On the other hand, the arbor is a bold frame that can easily become a focal point in this garden. The trees too, provide solid structure. But the biggest showstopper of all: that beautiful stream. It curves around the perimeter, providing harmonic framework and a natural border for the garden, beginning with the jasmine trim.

Evaluate

Now that we know what the key elements are, we can make an objective evaluation of each piece (table 2-1).

WHAT'S KEY	WHAT'S GREAT	THE REST
Stream	Flowers	Weeds, fallen leaves
Arbor	Birdbath	Crack in the birdbath
Trees	Birds	Ferns and hostas

Table 2-1

Notice that the third column isn't called "bad." The elements in the last column could detract or they could be neutral. Ferns and hostas aren't bad—they're just not as important as the things in the first two columns.

To take this a step further, we can give each element points so that we understand how each piece impacts the whole garden. By using points in our evaluation, we will be able to cleanly track how we rejuvenate this garden.

Should we evaluate everything in the garden with equal measure? Certainly not. The stream plays a much more important role than the birdbath. You might have noticed that all the "key elements" have one crucial thing in common: they provide structure. Key elements are worth more to this garden than anything else. The "great" elements are ornamental. Wonderful to have, but without the structure they're discombobulated and less meaningful. After the key elements and the great elements, everything else is a stack of wildcards.

- With that in mind, we might approach our evaluation like this:
- Key elements are worth a maximum of 20 points each
- Great elements are worth a maximum of 10 points each
- The rest can range anywhere from -3 to +3 points
- Now, let's apply this system to our garden (table 2-2).

WHAT'S KEY	PTS	WHAT'S GREAT	PTS	THE REST	PTS
Stream	+20	Flowers	+7	Weeds, fallen leaves	-5
Arbor	+14	Birdbath	+5	Crack in the birdbath	-2
Trees	+18	Birds	+10	Ferns and hostas	+3
Subtotal:	52	*Subtotal:*	22	*Subtotal:*	-4

Table 2-2

Add up the subtotals of all three columns, and the final number is 70. The stream contributed the most to the score, while the weeds were the biggest detractor.

The Palmer Code [Francis Palmer MD]

Focus

Our evaluation complete, we understand the key elements, the great elements and how they all contribute to the big picture. Now we know where to put our focus. As long as the focus is on the best parts, the rest fades into the background.

To revitalize this garden, we focus on all the things in the first two columns, but we must do so methodically. Build the great things around the key elements that provide structure and you'll have a magnificent creation. With this in mind, you can take action:

- Move the flowers so that they follow the pattern of the stream or build off the structure of the arbor
- Group similar flowers together to add even more structure
- Arrange moss or creeping plants on the birdbath to camouflage the crack
- Remove the weeds and anything else that gets in the way
- Water, nurture, and preen

With a little attention, the natural beauty of the garden comes forth. Most of the changes listed above will have an instant affect. The last one, nurturing your garden, will actually have the most dramatic affect over time. That's when the flowers double and triple in volume, so that an observer may think that they're what make this garden great. That's true to an extent, but you know that structure played a critical role.

Structure + Ornament = Masterpiece

Now that we've revitalized this garden, let's see how the scores might have changed (table 2-3):

WHAT'S KEY	PTS	WHAT'S GREAT	PTS	THE REST	PTS
Stream	+20	Flowers	+10	Weeds, fallen leaves	0
Arbor	+14	Birdbath	+7	Crack in the birdbath	0
Trees	+18	Birds	+10	Ferns and hostas	+3
Subtotal:	52	*Subtotal:*	27	*Subtotal:*	3

Table 2-3

Now our garden has a number assessment of 82. Significant change from 70, don't you think?

It's easy to look at a garden and know that you can nurture and cultivate it to take it to a higher level. Even though the garden is made up of living things, it has no ego. The most effective way to achieve greatness is to shed the ego. It just gets in the way. This is a belief that falls in step with most spiritual teachings throughout time. The Bible, for example, celebrates physical beauty most notably in the book of Psalms.

> • • •
> ## "The most effective way to achieve greatness is to shed the ego."
> • • •

This simple, yet effective, garden exercise demonstrates how the *Palmer Code* elements can be used to create real change and real improvements in your appearance and your life. Think of your life as the garden.

What Your Number Can Do for You

When you determine your *Palmer Code number*, you take control. You don't have to resign yourself to fate; instead you create your own present and future. Think of it as art. It's important to set aside the ego and take an objective look in order to create the vision.

Leonardo Da Vinci hungered for knowledge in the world around him and even within himself. He experimented with things like writing backwards, constantly pushing the limits and stepping away from the familiar. If you're willing to depart from your usual beauty routine—the same make-up and clothes—and take a fresh, scientific approach to the *outer you*, you give yourself a chance at real metamorphosis. Da Vinci applied his creativity to math, science, art and inventions that stepped outside the boundaries of his time. You don't have to have Leonardo Da Vinci's brain to visualize your ideal self, but you can use a similar approach in combining art and science. I've done the scientific research for you, so the hard part is already finished.

My goal, my professional mission as a plastic and cosmetic surgeon, is to give people the ability and power to know there's a vast diversity of things they can do to make themselves look better. I don't want you to simply know *your number*. I want to empower you with the information to help you create something amazing.

As a point of reference, let's begin by taking a look at the *Palmer Code number* distribution within the general population .

The Number of the Common Man

Whenever you examine the population at large, it's common to use the bell-shaped curve as a rule-of-thumb estimation. The bell curve is a mathematical distribution that shows what's rare and what's typical with regards to a specific trait. The bulk of the population lands right in the middle and people with rare qualities or relatively few are represented in the narrower bottom flare on both sides of the bell.

So where does that put the average person in terms of the *Palmer Code?* If we take *face numbers* as an example, the vast majority of people have a *Palmer Code face number* that falls between 60 and 75. Stretch a little above average, and you're in the category of "Attractive." Attractive people have *numbers* from 76-84. People with *numbers* from 85-94 are stunningly beautiful and those at the highest end, with *numbers* from 95-100, are very few and far between. Marilyn Monroe, Audrey Hepburn and Angelina Jolie are good examples of people in this category. They're beauties that are rare and memorable. They become icons. I call them "Star Quality Beautiful".

[Francis Palmer MD]　The Palmer Code

Here the bell-shaped curve (table 2-4) shows the *distribution* of beauty among the general population. The bottom line shows *Palmer Code numbers* ranging from 1 all the way to a perfect 100 (Brad Pitt and Angelina Jolie). The left side of the bell-shaped curve shows the percentage of the population in each category: average, attractive, stunningly beautiful, or star-quality beautiful. We also see that half of the population has a below-average face number and half are people with above-average face numbers.

Palmer Code Numbers from Low to Highest

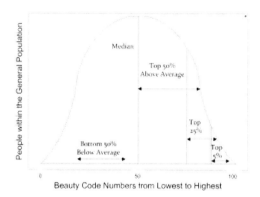

Table 2-4

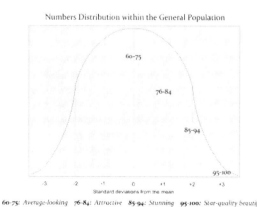

Table 2-5

The Palmer Code   [Francis Palmer MD]

Placing the distribution of *face numbers* into the bell-shaped curve (Table 2-5), you could say that the vast majority—or the average person—is *average looking*, with *face numbers* between 60 and 75. People in the "attractive" category, with numbers between 76-84, occupy a narrower percentage. The stunners with *face numbers* from 85-94 are rarer still and that very tiny percentage of the population who qualifies as star-quality beautiful with numbers between 95-100: those are the rarest of the rare. You can see on the bell-shaped curve just how uncommon that level of beauty truly is. Think about it. When's the last time you saw somebody as beautiful as Halle Berry walking down the street?

As you go through the *Palmer Code* steps, you'll get an understanding of where you fit in the bell-shaped curve. You'll also find out how you can change so that you fall closer to that coveted bottom right spectrum. *The Palmer Code* is not just about your face, body, *inner you, outer you* or your *whole number*. There's little value in knowing you're an 83. The power is in knowing *why* you're an 83, *understanding* the key elements and *taking educated steps* to enhance *your number*. This book is a transformative experience on many levels, from discovering exactly where you stand to finding out how you can improve. I'm inviting you to try a new, precise and motivating way to look at yourself.

Why should you care about the *Palmer Code* and what it has to offer? Why would you want to know *your number* or learn how it could be improved? I think the answer is quite simple. It's human nature to seek improvement, that's why man went to the moon, explored the heavens and has made technological advancements to improve our quality of life. I believe that if asked "would you rather look better or worse", the vast majority of people would choose better because it somehow just makes sense.

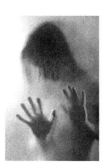

Chapter 3:
The Palmer Code and Your Number

During the course of my practice, when I first devised the number system, I reflexively analyzed people and determined their *face* or *body numbers*. I'd realized I'd come across something meaningful and was fascinated by the way the system proved itself, over and over thousands of times, allowing me to improve the appearance of my patients in the operating room. After a while however, I trained myself to shut it off because it felt like an invasion. I no longer analyzed people unless they asked me, to do so, during a medical consultation. But people do ask me. In fact they ask all the time: "Hey doc, *what's my number?*"

We live in a competitive society. Whether we like it or not, an 86 has advantages a 74 doesn't. More than $12 billion were spent last year in the U.S. on plastic surgery procedures and non-invasive beauty treatments. Many billions more were spent on makeup, clothing, hairstyles, exercise equipment, gym memberships, nutritional supplements, diet books, skin care, beauty products and non-medical beauty enhancements. People are interested in their looks.

I understand that compulsion; believe me, beauty's my business, but I wish I could stand up and address the population at large. I would tell everyone to stop, to put away those credit cards for just a minute and to hold off on spending one more penny until they really understand where that money can best be spent. A frenzied approach is at best ineffective and often is just plain madness. The true reality is that from knowledge comes insight and with that, the power to affect meaningful change.

The Palmer Code [Francis Palmer MD]

Beauty Equations

Some of what we'll be discussing in this book entails the mechanics of physical beauty: How to fine-tune your physical self to bring the best of you into focus. But before we do that it's important to examine the other components that contribute to your *Palmer Code number*.

The *Palmer Code* is an equation that takes into account both the *outer you* and the *inner you*. The *outer you* is what you see in the mirror. It's also what others see and process into "first impressions" during that initial split second when they encounter someone new. The *inner you* is your essence, the light and energy which you emanate. It's your personality, your presence and your power. Once you explore these components you'll realize that your beauty is not determined by the nose you don't like or the ears you think are too big. It's far more complex, individual, and quite frankly, wonderful than any one of those things.

Outer You (60%) + Inner You (40%) = Your Number (100%)

In the context of first impressions and superficial encounters, the *outer you* comprises 60% of *your number*. Like it or not, it's human nature and hard-wired into our brains that way. Of course for long-term and platonic situations the focus becomes the *inner you*, but even in the context of basic attraction, it's a mistake to discount the *inner you* component, because an increase or decrease of 40% is pretty significant. If you start with a number of 83 but your inner light takes that impression to a 93, you've jumped from attractive to stunning on the bell curve.

Here's an example. Two thirty-something women are in a bar. At first glance, both have *outer you numbers* of 92. As we sit and continue to observe both women it becomes clear that one woman has a pleasant personality with open body language that announces she is both friendly and confident. The other woman however appears sullen, closed and ill-tempered with body language that says "stay away." Now, how would you rate their *numbers*? The mean-spirited woman will no doubt be perceived as less attractive because of her negative personality (perceived because we're all too afraid to go and speak with her) and body language. The end result? Her *number* will go down.

The Whole Number Components

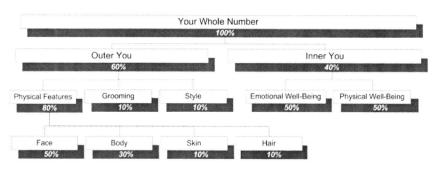

Table 3-1

As you can see, there are many factors that feed into your *whole number* (table 3-1). Let's take a closer look at those.

First, the *outer you* is made up of components that fit into three main categories: physical features, grooming and style. The equation looks like this:

Physical Features (80%) + Grooming (10%) + Style (10%) = Outer you (100%)

Clearly, your physical features count most toward your outer appearance. I'm sure you already knew that intuitively. Hygiene (included in grooming) and clothes (part of style) can dramatically improve or hinder appearance, but not to the extent of physical attributes. However we have all seen Pygmalion transformations where impeccable grooming and style has revealed a diamond in the rough. These are supporting—but nevertheless still quite important—factors that contribute to *your number*.

The Palmer Code [Francis Palmer MD]

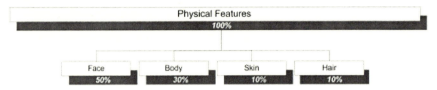

Table 3-2

Breaking the equation down, we see that your physical features are composed of your face, body, skin, and hair (table 3-2).

Face (50%) + Body (30%) + Skin (10%) + Hair (10%) = Physical Features (100%)

When it comes to analyzing the physical features category, the face accounts for 50% of the equation, the body 30%, skin 10% and hair 10%. You may be wondering why the face plays such an important role in the equation, contributing substantially more points than the body. That's because we are accustomed to looking at faces. In fact I believe we are genetically wired this way.

Studies have shown that an infant is able to recognize its mother's face at a very early age. Similarly, babies in these studies cried, showed fear and anxiety when scary masks were placed over otherwise familiar faces. We, as humans, are hard-wired to look at faces and it seems we are similarly wired to gravitate towards attractive faces. For this reason, your face contributes a higher percentage to the equation in the physical features category than anything else, including your body. Here again, you probably already knew this intuitively.

> • • •
> **"We are genetically wired to look at faces."**
> • • •

This casts an important light on issues of body weight. An overweight woman might have a very pretty face, as the fat plumps up the cheeks in just the right places, though modern society perceives too much fat on the body as less attractive. Yet in that crucial moment, that split second when first impressions occur and the subconscious provides an assessment of that *Palmer Code number*, it's the face that contributes most to basic primal attraction.

Skin and hair play a supporting role in the equation. Beautiful skin and hair can add points to *your number*, but they factor in to a much lesser degree than things like beautiful cheeks, full lips, or an hourglass figure. Nevertheless, as we will discuss later on in this book, because skin and hair are malleable ingredients in your appearance, they will become important players when you are seeking ways to increase *your number*.

"It's essential to maintain good health in order to maintain your number."

A Closer Look at the Outer you

Remember that imaginary woodland garden? It's time to apply some of those principles to human physical features. By examining the face, body, skin and hair individually, we take the first steps toward defining the key elements, as well as the features that are great or neutral. This is similar to identifying the parts of the garden—flowers, trees, stream and so on.

We'll start with the feature that comprises the lion's share of the number for physical features: the face.

Facial Components

Shape

A face may be square, round, rectangular or heart-shaped. For men, square or rectangular shapes are considered most attractive; for women, the softer lines of an oval or heart shaped face are preferable.

The Palmer Code [Francis Palmer MD]

Forehead shape, slope and position

A forehead may vary in length or prominence. The ideal angle for the forehead as it meets the nose is 140 degrees.

Eyebrow

Women have ideally shaped brows when they are tapered and arched in relation to the upper edge of the eye socket. For men, the ideal is more full and flat in position.

Eyes

Contributing factors include shape, color and presence of extra skin and fatty tissue. The eyes are a significant contributor to facial structure. They are also the first to show signs of aging. Women's eyes look best when they appear open, well defined and are free of excess skin or fatty tissue. For men, ideal eyes tend to be smaller, with more skin obstructing the eyelid creases. Only with advanced skin fullness does this become a beauty detraction for men.

Cheeks

The tissue of the face literally hangs from the cheeks, which makes the cheeks crucial to facial structure. Female cheeks are ideally shaped when full and round, while men look best with cheeks that are more narrow and angular.

Nose

Look at size, shape, the tip and nostrils. The nose should be sleek and unobserved so that the cheeks, eyes and lips are what attracts attention. Perfect noses actually add little to the overall facial score, but a nose that is too long, too short, too wide, or too crooked can detract.

Lips

Lips are ideally shaped when they are full and pouty. Beautiful lips have the power to soften the lower half of the face. A weak chin or imperfect nose can be balanced by full lips. The upper lip should be no more than 75% the size and fullness of the lower lip. Another way to say this would be the ideal size of the lower lip is 1.33 times that of the upper lip.

Chin

When examining the chin, look at size and shape. The chin is the anchor of the face when seen in profile. A weak chin will make the face appear relatively feminine; while a strong, square-shaped chin imparts a ruggedly masculine appearance to the face.

Jaw line

One of the most important aspects of the jaw line is the degree of its flare. Imagine that the chin forms a triangle with the ears. The chin is the apex, the jawline forms the sides and a line between the ears becomes the base. Wider angles (more flared) are generally seen as more attractive, however extremely wide angles create a masculine look, preferable only for men.

Neck

Look at the shape in relation to the jaw line and chin. Also examine the length: swan-like is beautifully feminine; muscular is masculine. Other important factors include the amount of excess skin, fat and the presence of lines and wrinkles.

Skin

The skin should be soft, supple and smooth with consistent color (pigmentation) while being free of wrinkles, blemishes and acne scars.

The Palmer Code [Francis Palmer MD]

So how much does each of the above facial features contribute overall? Bearing in mind the woodland garden and how structure helped us to determine key elements, take a guess as to what might be the most important features of the face. For now, I'll let you think about it, but I'll give you a hint: you might be surprised by the star facial feature. We'll take a much closer look in "Chapter 4: The Palmer Code for the Face."

The Body

Overall shape

Rectangular, square, round, pear. For both men and women, long, lean, rectangular body shapes are perceived as more healthy, fit and attractive.

Torso/leg shape

A v-shaped torso is perceived as ruggedly masculine. For women, an hourglass shape reflects timeless feminine beauty, as remembered in such legends as Marilyn Monroe, Raquel Welch and Sophia Loren.

Torso/leg ratio

Men look balanced when the legs and torso are close to a 50/50 ratio. This means that their body appears to be roughly half head/torso and half hips/legs. Women, on the other hand, look best when the head/torso ratio is lower compared to the hips and legs. Simply put, the longer the legs the better. In reality, women look best with a head/torso to hip/leg ratio of 40/60 to 35/65.

Shoulders, arms, chest, legs, and hips

Consider size, shape, girth and tone. Men look best when muscular but not bulky; women look best with lengthy, toned muscles.

[Francis Palmer MD] **The Palmer Code**

Skin (overall)

Degree of firmness and tone (loose skin)

Texture

Change in pigmentation

Wrinkles and folds

Excess fatty tissue

Blemishes and contour defects (scars, acne pock marks)

Hair

Amount/fullness of hair

Hair/forehead ratio (degree of thinning)

Texture

Style

Color

Grooming

This category can be divided into hairstyle, makeup and hygiene. I know you're wondering, "How much does my hairstyle have to do with it?" The answer is, a great deal.

Let's imagine two 41 year-old women. Suppose they have similar faces and bodies, but one woman has a hairstyle that compliments her face, while the second has a hairstyle that disregards facial structure. You may have already guessed where I'm going with this by now. The second woman will have a lower overall *number* because her hairstyle diverts focus away from, instead of complementing, her face.

The type of hairstyle you choose–one that's based on a scientific analysis of the shape of your face–can significantly affect *your number*. The next several chapters examine facial structure in detail. It might be worthwhile for you to go over these carefully before you go in for your next haircut.

31

Style

This category can be divided into clothing, color, and accessories. I'm sure it's no surprise that certain clothes make you feel more beautiful and therefore better than others. You've heard the term "the clothes make the man". The right color and style of clothing will improve your number just as surely as a horrendous set of clothing will decrease it. A unique sense of style can also convey a sense of personality, which reflects the *inner you*.

You may already know that colors and cuts can change the perception of your body. Consider the torso/leg ratio, as mentioned under "The Body" above. If a woman's body does not reflect the 40/60 torso/leg ratio, she can still create that look in the way she styles her clothes. The same is true for a man. Sometimes a simple matter of tucking in the shirt can mean the difference in a man's perceived 50/50 torso/leg ratio.

The Inner You

The *inner you*, which makes up 40% of your *Palmer Code number*, is divided equally between emotional and physical well-being, each of which has numerous contributing factors reflecting the complexities of our modern lives (table 3-3).

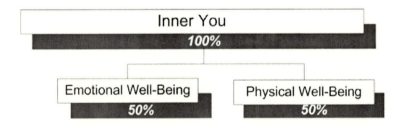

Table 3-3

[Francis Palmer MD] **The Palmer Code**

The *inner you* is affected by many differing factors. Here are just a few:

Relationships (at work, at home, with God, the universe, or a higher existence)

Your overall physical health

Your emotional health

Your feelings of self worth

How you fit in and contribute to society

Stress levels (work, home)

Attitude towards life (you, other people, the world)

These factors contribute to your state of mind, your health, and your spirit. They reflect out into the world in the form of personality and sense of peace.

Suppose two 43 year-old men each have *numbers* of 88. One man is in good overall health, exercises regularly and eats a sensible diet. The other man doesn't exercise and has the early signs of increased blood pressure and cholesterol. How long do you think it will be before the second man sees his *number* start to decrease? Over time, the hypertension effects his energy level and mood, perhaps even resulting in the occasional headache; the lack of exercise makes him feel slow and out of shape. He may begin to feel less confident than he used to and as a result he might be less outgoing. His *number* declines little by little, in incremental but inevitable degrees.

We all know that when we have a cold or flu, we feel lousy and usually look pretty lousy too. Our physical and emotional health can have a very real impact on the way we look. It's essential to maintain good health in order to maintain *your number*.

We'll go into further detail in a later chapter devoted to the *inner you*.

The Palmer Code   [Francis Palmer MD]

Bringing it all Together

Add together the individual components that make up the *outer you* and the *inner you,* and you understand your *Palmer Code number:* (table 3-4)

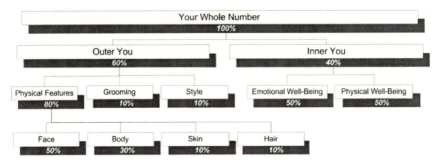

Table 3-4

These, essentially, are all the elements in your garden of life. Each piece acts as a key to unlock your *Palmer Code number.*

Over the next several chapters, we'll take a look at how to get the most of each piece, with the greatest focus on the one element that we are hardwired to respond to on a primal level: the face.

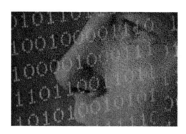

Chapter 4:
The Palmer Code for the Face

At the core of the *Palmer Code* are the secret, ideal patterns that define human beauty. Understanding them and how they relate to you will allow the full potential of your appearance to be revealed. You'll literally have a map for unlocking your true hidden beauty.

In this chapter you will learn what have, until now, been my trade secrets. Algorithms I've used thousands of times to get stunningly beautiful results for my patients. This same information will help you determine your own *face number* and with that understanding comes a clear picture of how to optimize your appearance using makeup, hairstyle, facial exercises, skin care, or any one of the many other facets of your facial appearance.

Facial Shapes

Before examining specific features, let's look at overall facial shape. Faces can be square, circular, oval, rectangular or heart-shaped (figures 4-2 to 4-7). Generally speaking, men look ruggedly handsome with more angular faces (rectangular or square). Women on the other hand do well with faces that are perceived as soft and full (oval or heart-shaped). Less pleasing, circular and triangular, shapes have foreheads that overshadow the cheeks, making the face appear top-heavy and out of proportion.

The Palmer Code [Francis Palmer MD]

Consider these examples of the various facial shapes:

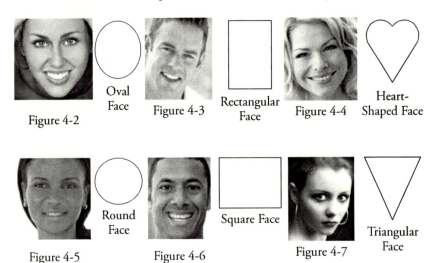

Figure 4-2 — Oval Face
Figure 4-3
Figure 4-4 — Rectangular Face
Figure 4-4 — Heart-Shaped Face
Figure 4-5 — Round Face
Figure 4-6
Figure 4-7 — Square Face
Figure 4-7 — Triangular Face

Face Shapes on Profile

Profiles (examples shown below) can be straight, curved inward (concave) or curved outward (convex). Profiles that are straight allow facial features to appear balanced and for this reason they are considered ideal. The concave profile (with a recessed midsection/cheek but prominent forehead/chin), or the convex profile (characterized by a prominent nose with recessed forehead and chin) both result in facial imbalance and are therefore less desirable.

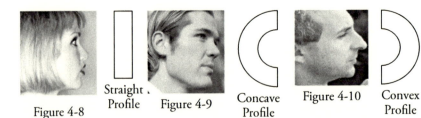

Figure 4-8 — Straight Profile
Figure 4-9
Figure 4-10 — Concave Profile
Figure 4-10 — Convex Profile

[Francis Palmer MD] **The Palmer Code**

The Sexes

Beauty features can be regarded as relatively masculine (angular, chiseled) or feminine (soft, round). I refer to these as being *gender-specific*. For example, if you're a man, the more masculine your features, the more handsome you are. The converse is also true. Women with more feminine features are regarded as more attractive.

Facial Features

Now let's take a closer look at specific facial features. Facial beauty is controlled and determined by three key facial features—the "big three," as I call them. Together they account for 92% of how attractive your face is perceived. And the most important element of these three may surprise you…

> **"The Palmer Code reveals the cheeks as the most important facial feature."**

It's the cheeks.

That's right. Although, as they say, the eyes are the "windows to the soul," they are not the most important feature of facial beauty. Not by a long shot. It's the cheeks.

The Big Three

- **Cheeks: 75 points**
  Full and round for women; narrow and angular for men

- **Eyebrows/Eyes: 10 points**
  Eyebrows high and arched for women; flat and low for men. Eyes larger (more open) for women with less upper lid skin.

- **Lips: 7 points**
  Full and plump with upper lip 75% as full as the lower lip for both sexes.

Total for the "big three" beauty features….**92 points** out of a possible 100.

The Palmer Code   [Francis Palmer MD]

From the information, presented above, you can see that the cheeks are the most aesthetically important feature of a youthful, beautiful face. Beauty's trigger point, they can literally cause an observer to perceive a face as being male, female, attractive, unattractive, youthful or aging. This one feature, when ideally shaped, is responsible for the major balance of facial beauty, a whopping 75% to be exact. Surprised? Don't be.

Think of it this way: the face literally hangs by the cheekbones, and if they are particularly well-shaped, they not only make you look beautiful today, they make it less likely that key facial areas will fall and sag with age. By defining the shape of your cheeks, you create a beauty focal point.

Not convinced? Try this simple exercise:

Making no expression, look into a mirror. Then do it again, but this time smile.

What happened? As you smile, the tissues of the mid-face (cheeks) are forced into a higher, more youthful and aesthetic position making your entire face look younger and more attractive. Why does this occur? Because smiling pushes the facial tissues back onto the cheeks, thereby allowing them to approach their ideal aesthetic shape.

It's simple. Smiling makes the entire face more beautiful. So be sure to smile for every photograph, especially as you grow older.

Calculating your Cheek Volume

Figure 4-11 shows ideally-shaped cheeks for women. To measure your cheek, look straight into a mirror and draw an imaginary vertical line through the pupil (vertical line in figure 4-11) down the front of your face. As you do this, you can feel where the cheekbone ends. Next, draw an imaginary horizontal line across from the bottom of the nostril (horizontal line in figure 4-11). The cheekbone should extend down the face to the point where these two imaginary lines intersect. That ideal volume will create

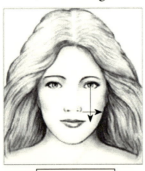

Figure 4-11

38

a cheek that's full and round, making the face look soft, youthful, feminine and more attractive.

Compare that to figure 4-12 that depicts ideally-shaped cheeks for men. Unlike those in beautiful women, ideal male cheeks are narrow and elevated higher from the face for a more angular rugged appearance.

Let's take a closer look and see exactly what the ideal male cheek shape looks like. Figure 4-12 uses the same imaginary lines that we used to calculate a woman's cheek, but the end result is a more narrow and angular looking cheek. Men, follow the same maneuver described above for women's cheeks, but this time the intersection point of the two imaginary lines is higher on the face (see arrow). This higher, narrow shaped cheek will give the face more angular, chiseled, relatively masculine good looks.

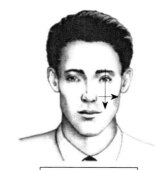

Figure 4-12

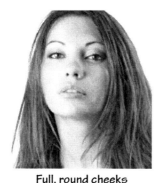

Full, round cheeks

Figure 4-13

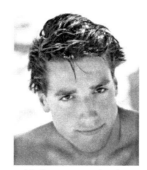

High, narrow cheeks

Figure 4-14

The Palmer Code   [Francis Palmer MD]

The Eyes and Eyebrows

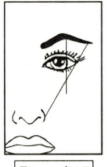

Figure 4-15

Together the eyebrows and eyes comprise the second most aesthetically important feature, representing 10% of facial beauty. For Eyebrows, the formula relies upon position and shape. Figure 4-15 shows the prototypical female eyebrow: club shaped, arching at a 45 degree angle to a peak and then tapering to a point. The peak intersects an imaginary vertical line along the outer iris, with the tapered section placed above the edge of the eye socket by about the width of your little finger.

Men, on the other hand, have much lower-placed, flat, fuller eyebrows without arching or tapering. The rest of the formula relies on key eye characteristics like an ideal almond shape, prominent eyelid crease and lack of excess fat and skin in both sexes.

Unusually colored eyes are another way to appear more attractive, as fans of Frank Sinatra and Elizabeth Taylor can attest.

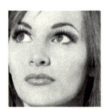

Figure 4-16

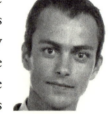

Figure 4-17

Figure 4-16 illustrates the ideally shaped female eyebrow and eye. The upper eyelid has a discernable crease with a soft gentle fold above it. Both the upper and lower eyelids are free of excess skin or fatty bulges that disrupt the soft gentle eyelid curvature. The ideal male brow (figure 4-17) is flat. The upper eyelid crease is far less visible and looks best with some fullness along their upper lid. This combination of eyebrow/eye characteristics is what is often called "bedroom eyes".

The Lips

Lips are the third most important facial feature, accounting for 7% of facial beauty, but are also the most commonly overlooked. Lips, when ideally shaped (figure 4-18), are full and plump, but the key formula for beautiful lips lies in the proportion between them. The upper lip should be roughly 75% as large as the lower, allowing the lower lip to look full with a pout. Ideal lips, like the ones in this photo, can camouflage a less-than-ideal nose or chin by drawing an observer's gaze and softening the entire lower face.

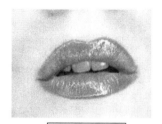

Figure 4-18

Remember, these three facial features will determine whether your face is perceived as young, old, male, female, beautiful or less so. Make sure you have a thorough understanding of their power before moving on to the rest of this chapter.

Ok let's take a look at the supporting cast of facial features, beginning with the nose.

The Nose

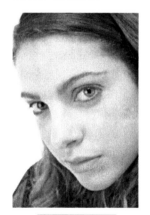

Figure 4-19

Ah, the perfect nose. There must be some kind of misunderstanding. It seems people obsess over their noses more than any other facial feature, and the statistics hammer that point home—rhinoplasty tops the list of plastic surgeries performed year after year. That fact not withstanding, I'm here to dispel the myth that the nose is a great contributor to facial beauty. In fact, I think of the nose as the Rodney Dangerfield of facial features because it literally "gets no respect."

Here's an example:

I recall a particularly gorgeous model that flew in from Paris, asking me to perform revision nasal surgery. I spent much of the consultation convincing her that her nose required very little work. Instead, it just

41

The Palmer Code [Francis Palmer MD]

needed to look more natural and not like it had nine prior operations. That's right, I said nine previous surgeries. She'd been so obsessed with making her nose symmetric and perfect that she had way too many surgeries (performed elsewhere, not by me). Sadly, each subsequent surgery made her nose look more unnatural, which came at the expense of her overall facial beauty.

So what's the deal, you ask? Why are hundreds of thousands of nose jobs done in this country every year if the nose isn't that important? The answer is simple. Many men and women see minor imperfections in their noses and think that the rest of us see the same thing…but we don't. **I am here to tell you today that the nose, as a beauty feature, is highly over-rated.**

The simple truth is, most people don't realize that they can be beautiful without having a perfect nose. Ideally, the nose should appear sleek and refined without major flaws that draw the observer's focus. When it comes to the nose, it's what isn't there that's important. If the nose has some "off" feature (a large hump, or a tip that's crooked, large, asymmetric, or over-rotated up/down) the nose draws unwanted attention to itself.

Attention on the nose means that the observer's gaze is distracted away from the "big three" beauty features (cheeks, eyes and lips). Definitely not what you want happening when someone's looking at your face.

On the contrary, when people look at you they should notice your cheeks first, then your eyebrows/eyes and then your lips……not your nose! Not ever.

Ideal noses do exist, and have some key aspects that include:

- 140 degree angle between the nasal bridge and the forehead
- The nasal tip should be rotated, from the upper lip, at an angle of 105 to 115 degrees
- The width ratio of the tip (top to base) is 1:3

While ideal is nice, it's definitely not required. In fact, you can look absolutely gorgeous with an average-looking nose that's gender specific and natural.

The take-away message is simple. No matter how you do it your nose only needs to look refined, without major flaws. It does not need to be perfect. You will never achieve beauty just because you have a perfect nose. Instead, a nose that is unobserved allows your "big three" beauty features to shine through and steal the show.

The Rest

Like the nose, the jaw line, neck, and chin add bonus points to the face after the big three features have been analyzed.

The Neck

First, let's look at the neck. Buried deep inside the neck is a small bone called the hyoid. If the hyoid is positioned high in the neck (the ideal position) it forms an angle of 90 degrees or less with the chin, giving the neck a slender, pleasing shape. But if the hyoid is lower in the neck, it forms an angle greater than 90 degrees, which makes the neck appear shallow, short, full and less attractive.

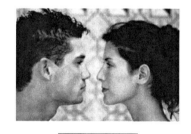

Figure 4-20

The ideal neck (figure 4-20) is elongated and swanlike in women but more muscular and powerful-looking in men. Excess fatty tissue and skin makes the neck appear less than ideal, causing a decrease in the *face number*.

The Jaw

The jaw line creates an aesthetic separation between the neck and chin, making it an integral part of facial shape and beauty. Flared jaw lines long associated with strength and masculinity are ideally male while smaller, softer jaw lines are better suited for women. See the effect of differently flared jaws illustrated below.

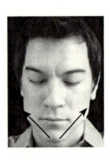

Figure 4-21 flared jaw line (wide angle)

The more flared the jaw line, the more masculine this feature becomes. Flared is a term that refers to how wide the angle is between the front of the chin and the back of the jaw.

The man's jaw in figure 4-21 has a wider angle while the man in figure 4-22 has one that is narrow. I think we all can agree that the man in figure 4-21 is more ruggedly handsome. The flared jaw is one of the reasons.

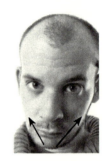

Figure 4-22 weaker jaw line (narrow angle)

The Chin

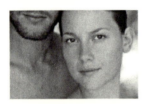

Figure 4-23

I'm sure it comes as no surprise that broad, squared chins are an ideal shape for men. Women however, appear more attractive with smaller, rounded chins. Regardless of gender, clefts and dimples add to attractiveness. Figure 4-23 portrays the difference between ideal male and female chin shapes.

The Skin

Quick, how many phrases can you recall that describe perfect skin? *Soft as a baby's bottom, peaches and cream complexion,* or how about *smooth as silk?* Most of us have an idea of what constitutes beautiful skin, and given that it's the body's largest organ, it should come as no

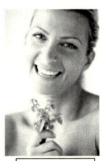

Figure 4-24

surprise that it's a rather important feature to our health. Ah, but it also plays a role in facial beauty.

Whatever the color or skin type, points are added for skin that is soft, smooth, firm and free of blemishes, pigment irregularity, laxity, scars, excess fat, lines and wrinkles.

How It All Comes Together

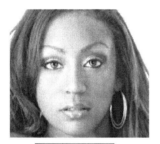

Figure 4-25

For the final assessment take an overall look and see if the facial features complement each other. In this face (figure 4-25), the cheeks, eyes, and lips first attract your attention, while the rest—the jaw line, chin, neck and skin—flow well. The nose, sleek and unobserved, fulfills its role allowing full appreciation of this face's beauty. This is an example of a well-balanced face with features that flow and complement each other.

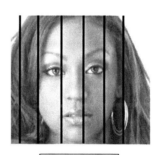

Figure 4-26

Next ask yourself if the face is fairly symmetric and balanced? Even though symmetry takes a backseat to ideally shaped features, there are some basic factors established by the ancient Greeks, embraced by Leonardo Di Vinci and others throughout history, that apply including the golden ratio Φ. The most notable, of which, are the rule of horizontal fifths (figure 4-26) and vertical thirds (figure 4-27).

Using the same face let's illustrate a fundamental principle of facial balance. The vertical lines show how an ideal face can be divided into five equal segments with each one approximately the width of one eye (figure 4-26).

Similarly, the face ideally can be divided in three equal vertical segments (figure 4-27).

The Palmer Code [Francis Palmer MD]

- Forehead—the upper third
- Mid-face—the middle third (eyes and cheeks)
- Lower face—the lower third (the lips and chin)

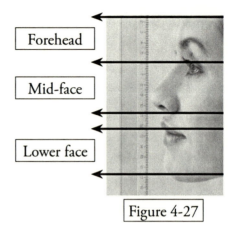

Figure 4-27

The lower third (the Lower-face) is further divided into a third for the upper lip and two-thirds for the lower lip and chin. Together these characteristics comprise the main tenets of facial symmetry and balance.

I imagine you might be a bit overwhelmed by all this information, but don't despair. It's OK to re-read this chapter several times in order to gain a thorough understanding of the beauty concepts that contribute to your *face number*. In the following chapters we'll go through how this knowledge can be used to not only calculate your own *face number*, but maximize it.

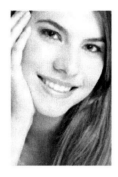

Chapter 5:
Your Own Face Number and the Big Three

Now it's time to apply some of this information to your own face.

In the last chapter we looked at three important keys to the *Palmer Code* for the face:

1. The cheeks—not the eyes—most influence the *Palmer Code face number*.
2. Both men and women look more beautiful when their features appear *gender-specific*.
3. The more ideal beauty features a person has, the higher the *Palmer Code face number*.

The individual components and their relevance to your *face number* can be expressed in the following formula:

Cheeks (75%) + Eyes (10%) + Lips (7%) + The Rest (8%) = Your Face Number (100%)

Because they are the stars of this show at 75% of your *face number*, we'll begin by analyzing your cheeks.

The Palmer Code [Francis Palmer MD]

How to Calculate Your Own Face Number

I recommend that you grab a pencil and stand in front of a mirror. Use the worksheet in "Appendix A: What's Your Number® Worksheet" at the end of this book to help you keep track as you move along through your analysis. Use the figures provided and choose the one that most closely matches your specific feature. If you feel that you are not quite an exact match, choose the one you most closely resemble and take an approximation of the corresponding point value. For example, if you feel that your cheeks are between the 65 and 60 point cheek figures, choose the one you most closely resemble. Let's say, it's the 65 cheeks. Give yourself the difference between 65 and 60, in this case 63 points. Use this analysis method, as you go through the remainder of this book for all features of the face and body that you'll be evaluating.

The Cheeks

I hope I hammered this point home in the previous chapters: the cheeks are the most aesthetically important of all the facial features. They alone control whether the face is perceived as male, female, youthful or less so. As you go through the following exercise, match your cheeks to those in the sample images that most closely resemble your own and make a note of the corresponding point value. In the off chance (very rare) that your cheeks are vastly asymmetric, evaluate each cheek independently and add the two numbers together, and then divide by two. This will result in a more accurate cheek number.

Let's get started.

Female Cheeks

The ideal cheek volume is full and round especially toward the front of the face. To get a sense of how full and round your cheeks are, compare yours to those in the following set of pictures (figures 5-2 through 5-9). It's best to assess your cheeks without smiling for an accurate score.

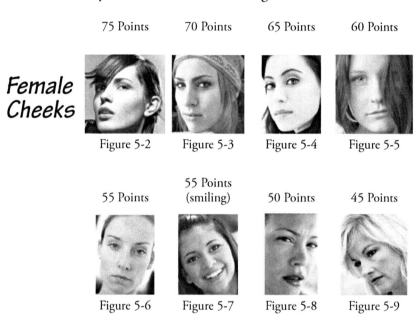

70 and 75-point cheeks are full and round. As the cheeks become flatter, folds develop between the nose and upper lip (nasolabial folds) and the point value decreases. Note that figure 5-7 represents cheeks with a fullness level of 55 points even though the woman appears to have fuller cheeks because she's smiling. For the purpose of your analysis, it's important to see beyond this to the basic structure of the cheeks. It does, however prove the point that a full smile will always round out the cheeks.

The Palmer Code [Francis Palmer MD]

Male Cheeks

Men, follow the same exercise to calculate your cheek volume and number. Match your cheeks to those in the images below (figures 5-10 to 5-16) and mark your cheek number accordingly.

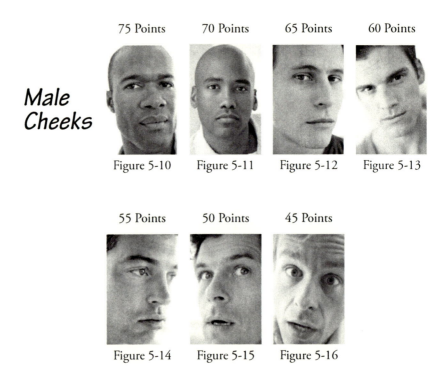

Male Cheeks

75 Points — Figure 5-10
70 Points — Figure 5-11
65 Points — Figure 5-12
60 Points — Figure 5-13
55 Points — Figure 5-14
50 Points — Figure 5-15
45 Points — Figure 5-16

[Francis Palmer MD] The Palmer Code

Eyes and Eyebrows (Eye Area)

The eyebrows and eyes **aren't** the leaders in facial beauty, but they play an important supporting role representing 10% of facial appearance. As you did with the cheeks, compare your eyebrows and eyes to the following examples and mark your score accordingly.

Female Eye Area:

For women, "almond" is the ideal aesthetic shape for the eyes, with the brows in a raised position arching and narrowing from the nose towards the ear. Compare yourself to figures 5-17 through 5-22 and record the corresponding value.

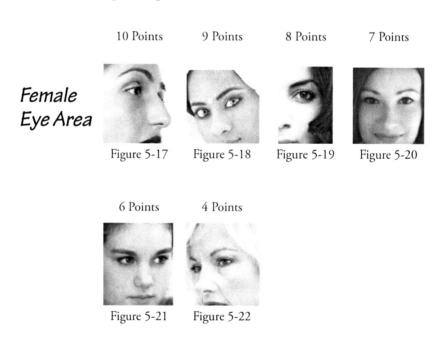

Female Eye Area

10 Points — Figure 5-17
9 Points — Figure 5-18
8 Points — Figure 5-19
7 Points — Figure 5-20
6 Points — Figure 5-21
4 Points — Figure 5-22

Eye area points decrease as the eyebrows fall from the ideal position, are an improper shape and excess skin and fat begins to accumulate along the upper or lower eyelids.

The Palmer Code [Francis Palmer MD]

Male Eye Area:

Men look best with lower placed, flatter, fuller brows with minimal arching or tapering and less prominent eyelid creases.

Take a look at figures 5-23 through 5-26 and compare yourself to those images in order to determine your score.

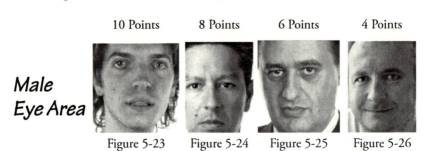

Male Eye Area

10 Points	8 Points	6 Points	4 Points
Figure 5-23	Figure 5-24	Figure 5-25	Figure 5-26

Points decrease as eyelid skin and fatty tissues accumulate.

Lips

Lips, the third most important feature, accounting for 7% of overall facial beauty are the one feature that's similar in both sexes. The lips, when ideally shaped, are full and plump but regardless of their fullness, the most important aspect is their ratio, of fullness, to one another. As long as the upper lip remains smaller than the lower lip the lips look balanced.

• • •

"Ideal lips, same for both sexes, when upper lip is ¾ the size of the lower lip."

• • •

The perfect relationship occurs when the upper lip is three-quarters the size of the lower lip giving them a slight pout; and pouty lips have a higher *number*.

Let's take a look at three sets of lips (figures 5-27 to 5-29) to illustrate this point. Which one do you think looks the best?

[Francis Palmer MD] The Palmer Code

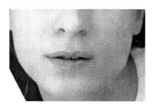
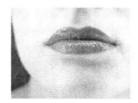
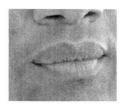

Figure 5-27 | Figure 5-28 | Figure 5-29

This upper lip is much thinner than the lower lip. | The upper lip is fuller but still smaller than the lower lip. | This upper lip is larger than the lower lip causing the lips to look out of balance.

If you answered the middle set of lips above, you are correct. They are both full and well proportioned.

Now match the following examples (figures 5-30 to 5-33) with your own lips, writing down the corresponding value.

Lips

7 Points | 6 Points | 5 Points | 3 Points

Figure 5-30a | Figure 5-31a | Figure 5-32a | Figure 5-33a

7 Points | 6 Points | 5 Points | 3 Points

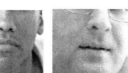

Figure 5-30b | Figure 5-31b | Figure 5-32b | Figure 5-33b

As the volume, of the lips, decreases the point value also decreases as it does with lips that out of proportion.

The Palmer Code [Francis Palmer MD]

Now go ahead and add the first three scores that you've received for your cheeks, eye area and lips. If ideal, they're worth up to 92 points. That's a staggering 92% of facial beauty. You just learned the secrets of the "big three" facial features that I often refer to as the *1-2-3 Beauty Punch*. Why? Because having beauty in these three areas of the face will make you a *knock-out*.

What's your *face number* so far? If you feel there's room for improvement, don't worry because in subsequent chapters you'll learn how you can improve your *face number* by bringing these elements to their full potential. Remember that every improvement begins first with knowledge and assessment. Without these, you have no direction and guidance on the most effective way to improve. OK, let's move on.

There are, as previously mentioned, other facial features that although less aesthetically important, do contribute to your *face number*, so let's go to the next chapter and calculate their value.

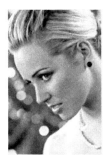

Chapter 6: Your Own Face Number for the Rest

You've calculated *your number* for the cheeks, eye area and lips, but keep your mirror handy because it's time to move on.

Skin

Ideally, women have skin that is soft, smooth, with a clear complexion and even skin tone. Men, the criteria are similar for you, except that your skin can appear more rugged. In short, skin should fade to the background and not attract notice.

Match your skin to figures 6-2 to 6-4 in order to determine your score.

Skin

2 Points	1 Point	0 Points
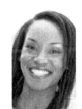	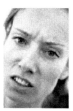	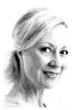
Figure 6-2a	Figure 6-3a	Figure 6-4a
2 Points	1 Point	0 Points
Figure 6-2b	Figure 6-3b	Figure 6-4b

The Palmer Code [Francis Palmer MD]

The facial skin should be free of sun damage, lines, wrinkles, spotty pigmentation, acnes scars, fatty tissue or loose skin which when present decrease the skin point value. ***In extreme cases of blemishes, scars, un-matched pigmentation, lines, wrinkles, and excess tissue, the skin can become a distraction causing additional points to be deducted from the *face number*.

Jaw Line, Neck, and Chin

Remember:

- The ideal jaw line for men is flared from the chin outward, whereas women look best with softer angles. Too sharp or too rounded, and the score drops.
- The ideal female neck is long and swan-like, and all necks look best when free of excess skin and fatty tissue.
- The chin should be balanced on profile.

Note, however that these features combined add only 2 points, so a lesser value won't cost you much.

Looking at figures 6-5 to 6-7, match yourself to the corresponding examples and record your value.

Jaw Line Neck & Chin

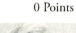

2 Points   1 Point   0 Points

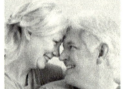

Figure 6-5a   Figure 6-6a   Figure 6-7

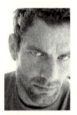
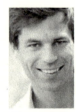

Figure 6-5b   Figure 6-6b

***In extreme cases of excess skin, fat, or shape distortion, a distraction may result in additional points being deducted from your face number.

Nose

Like the other facial features in this chapter, the nose is worth very few points and ideally shouldn't attract attention to itself and away from your face. Use figures 6-8 to 6-10 to help you determine your score.

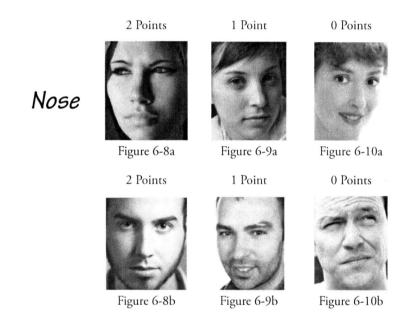

*Figure 6-9a has a bump on the bridge and a long nasal tip. Figure 6-10a has a long nose with wide (bulbous) tip cartilage and flared nostrils.

*Figure 6-9b has a long nose with thick tip cartilages. Figure 6-10 b has a crooked nose, flared nostrils and a wide, bulbous nasal tip.

***There are numerous reasons that a nose may receive less than the ideal 2 points. If there is some aspect, of the nose, (very large tip, large hump on bridge, very crooked, asymmetric tip, severely flared nostrils, over-operated look) that causes a major distraction to an observer

The Palmer Code [Francis Palmer MD]

looking at the face, this will result in 0 points for the nose and may even result in further points being deducted from the *face number*.

Overall Flow

If you scored well up until now, chances are your face has a nice overall flow with features that appear balanced and well-placed. This means your face has no significantly distracting qualities. Take a look at Figures 6-11 to 6-13 that are examples of overall flow. Compare yourself to these and record the appropriate points.

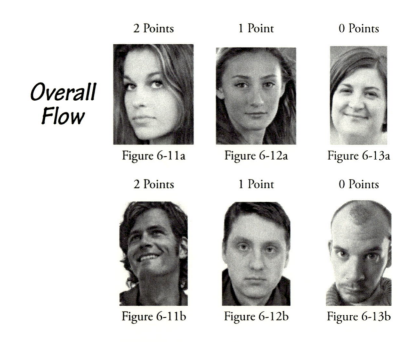

*Figure 6-12a has thin lips and a bit of a wide nasal tip. Figure 6-13a has a long nose, low eyebrows, excess skin of the upper eyelids, flat cheeks, deep nasolabial folds and thin lips.

***Figure 6-12b has flat cheeks and a thin upper lip. Figure 6-13b has low eyebrows, excess skin of the upper eyelids, a long nose with flared nostrils and a bulbous tip, flat cheeks, thin lips, small chin and weak jawline angle.

[Francis Palmer MD]   The Palmer Code

The skin, nose, jaw/chin/neck and overall flow can add up to a maximum of 8 points. Tally your score and then add that to your points for the "big three" facial features and you have your *Palmer Code Face Number*, or *face number* for short.

Big Three (92%) + The Rest (8%) = Your Face Number (100%)

Now that you've calculated your *face number*, get ready to take it to a whole new level. This is the equivalent of evaluating your garden space and planning a strategy for your metamorphosis. By understanding what's most important, you create focus where it counts.

But first, let's put your new method of analysis to the test. What's their *face number?* Use what you've learned so far to practice calculating the *face numbers* for the following set of face photos (figures 6-14 to 6-19). I have included an answer key at the end of this chapter for you to check your accuracy.

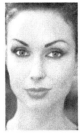

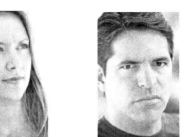

Figure 6-14   Figure 6-15   Figure 6-16

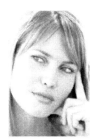
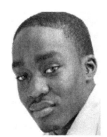
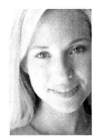

Figure 6-17   Figure 6-18   Figure 6-19

59

| | The Palmer Code | [Francis Palmer MD]

What's Their *Face Number* Answer key: 100 points possible

Figure 6-14: **97**

Cheeks 75; Eye Area 10; Lips 5 (-2 thin upper lip); Nose 1 (-1 wide tip); 6 out of 6 for all remaining supporting factors.

Figure 6-15: **80**

Cheeks 65; Eye Area 5 (-5 for low brows and excess upper lid skin); Lips 4 (-3 for thin upper lip); Nose 1 (-1 wide tip); Skin 2; Chin/Neck/Jaw Line 2; Overall Flow 1 (-1 lip and nose distract).

Figure 6-16: **82**

Cheeks 62; Eye Area 7 (-3 low brows); Lips 5 (-2 thin upper lip); 8 for all supporting factors.

Figure 6-17: **95**

Cheeks 72; Eye Area 8 (-2 low brows); Lips 7; 8 for all supporting factors.

Figure 6-18: **88**

Cheeks 70 (-5 in this case because they are too full and round, not narrow); Eye Area 10, Lips 4 (-3 upper lip larger than lower lip); Nose 0 (-2 wide, flared nostrils, wide tip); Skin 2; Chin/Neck/Jaw Line 2; Overall Flow 0 (-2 lips and nose distract).

Figure 6-19: **92**

Cheeks 70; Eye Area 9 (-1 low brows); Lips 6 (-1 thin upper lip); Nose 1 (-1 wide tip); 6 for remaining supporting factors.

Finally, I'd like to make a brief comment about *famous faces.* These are the *beautiful people, celebrities, royalty and fashionistas* that we can't seem to get enough of these days. Brad Pitt, Angelina Jolie, Jennifer Anniston, George Clooney just to name a few. If you've been wondering about the *face numbers* of the rich and famous and where some of them fit within the *Palmer Code,* you can see the *face number* of your favorite celebrity or try out your new skills by visiting our website http://www.whatsyournumbernews.com

Now that you've had some fun learning and calculating *face numbers*, it's time for you to learn how to harness this new knowledge and power to increase your own *face number*.

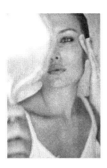

Chapter 7: Unlocking Your Face's Beauty Potential

Have you noticed something? The way you look definitely counts in the world and I don't mean that in the way you may be thinking. What I mean is, the way you look counts to the most important person in the world: you.

You've learned some important keys to the *Palmer Code*, but in order to make a transformation you must understand how this information applies to you. The following exercise is most effective if you write down your answers. So take a moment to grab a pencil. Go ahead. I'll wait. Got it? OK, let's go.

Exercise One

Imagine this: Suppose you have an important engagement—a business meeting, a meeting with your child's teacher, or perhaps you're going to attend a friend's wedding. Fix the scenario in your mind and take note of how you feel as you enter through a set of doors to greet the person or persons you plan to meet.

Now you see the other party and they see you. But suppose that just before you are about to shake hands or hug, you glance in the mirror and discover a wart on the tip of your nose. A giant, staring, knob in the style of the Wicked Witch of the West wart. You've already been spotted so it's too late to duck out of the meeting.

The Palmer Code   [Francis Palmer MD]

OK. Wart in place, you shake hands or hug (depending on who you're meeting) and then you continue into that important engagement. Go ahead, picture it and then ask yourself the following questions:

1. On a scale of one to ten, ten being the highest, what is your level of confidence?

   _____

2. Did your posture change after you glanced in the mirror? If so, how?

   _____

   _____

   _____

   _____

3. Are you able to completely focus on the business at hand?

   _____

   _____

4. Does the wart impact the way you present yourself in the meeting? How?

   _____

   _____

   _____

   _____

5. Would you say you're more relaxed than usual, or more tense?

   _____

   _____

For most of us, we will have a different experience if we sally forth warted as opposed to wartless. Some may even find a way to ditch the meeting altogether. Hang on to the sensations you've just experienced for just a moment, then move on to Exercise Two.

[Francis Palmer MD] **The Palmer Code**

Exercise Two

OK, back at the scene of that important engagement. Now imagine that it's not you who has a wart on the tip of your nose. Suppose that wart is sitting on the nose of the person you've just greeted.

1. Compared to the previous scenario, how do you feel about talking to someone who's got a wart on the nose?

    _____

    _____

    _____

2. On a scale of one to ten, ten being the highest, what is your level of confidence?

    _____

3. Did your posture change after you saw that poor warty person? If so, how?

    _____

    _____

    _____

4. Are you able to completely focus on the business at hand?

    _____

    _____

5. Does that wart impact the way you present yourself in the meeting? How?

    _____

    _____

    _____

6. Would you say you're more relaxed than usual, or more tense?

    _____

    _____

    _____

The Palmer Code [Francis Palmer MD]

Chances are, while you might have been distracted when you first noticed that wart, you feel much less disturbed than when the thing was attached to your own nose. During the course of your interaction, probably you would take note of the wart and then just continue about your business. And depending on how engaging your friend or colleague is, you may even forget about the wart from time to time and get lost in what he or she is saying.

So what's the point (so to speak)? It's simple. When your appearance has shifted from its baseline, there is one person in the world who cares the most about it: you. That wart on the tip of your nose changed what you perceive as your baseline appearance, that is, *how you are used to seeing yourself.* And while others take note, they rarely care about it as much as you do.

Exercise Three

Let's take this situation one step further. Forget about the wart. Now before you go into your important engagement, you check the mirror and are astonished to see that you look uncommonly attractive today! You are smoking hot! Things that you once might have called flaws in your appearance—that extra fold below your chin; the birthmark in the shape of the Texas Lone Star, your elongated earlobes—are diminished. Suppose your "usual" flaws are magically erased and what you see staring back from the mirror is the absolute best version of you. You see those bright, beautiful eyes, the chiseled bone structure, and the inevitable smirk that goes along with realizing just how devastatingly fabulous you look.

Feel it, hang onto it, then continue on to your appointment with this in mind.

1. On a scale of one to ten, ten being the highest, what is your level of confidence?

_____

[Francis Palmer MD] **The Palmer Code**

2. Did your posture change after you glanced in the mirror? If so, how?

_____

_____

_____

_____

3. Are you able to completely focus on the business at hand?

_____

_____

_____

_____

4. Does being a vision of the sublime affect the way you present yourself in the meeting? How?

_____

_____

_____

_____

5. Would you say you're more relaxed than usual, or more tense?

_____

_____

I'd be willing to wager that if we watched a DVD recording of both Warted You and Ideal You, we would find a significant difference in the way you present yourself and in the way you interact with others. Chances are these differences would be noticeable *even if all we played back was the sound*, and couldn't even see whether or not you were sporting the wart.

I'd also be willing to bet that of the three exercises above, the depth of your emotional response ranked the least for step two, when the wart was on someone else's nose. Why? Because it's not you! The way others look matters less to you than the way you look.

The Palmer Code [Francis Palmer MD]

Exercises one and three reflect a simple matter of confidence. Living your ideal appearance makes you feel good. It has an impact in the way you see yourself, and therefore it impacts the way you interact with others.

Baseline

Think of your beauty ideal as a kind of recipe. You are using the same ingredients as everyone else and maybe even the very same ingredients you've already been using yourself, but you may need to add a pinch of this or a dash of that in order to enhance the best flavors of that recipe.

In the previous chapters, you established your baseline by calculating *your number*. Understanding *your number* is the first step to reaching your full potential and by establishing a clear, objective assessment of this baseline, you can improve upon it. What's the result? It means living *every single day* in that ideal, sublime you. And guess what: You start now.

Makeup by the Numbers

Women, for most of you makeup can be an extremely valuable tool for maximizing your *face number*. In fact, you are already using it. But the question is, are you using it to your best advantage? Take a moment to consider how much time, money and effort you put into your makeup. Do you have an overall goal when applying it? What are the areas where you focus most of your attention? Do you have a broad collection of items that you rarely use?

Creating the ideal face should take very little time and require only a few key items. Your makeup should be fresh, not more than six months old, using hues that match your skin tone. As a general rule, women tend to look best with a natural look, using very light makeup during daylight hours and perhaps a bit more drama in the evening. You can, of course, experiment with color in eye shadows that coordinate with clothing and hair, but for the most part, build a kit that reflects your natural skin tones. Be aware that your hair is less important than your skin when it comes to matching makeup color. Concealer and blush form the basic structure for

68

your facial appearance, so take your time when selecting these products. You'll want to match your flesh tone as closely as possible, using products that blend evenly and feel light on your skin.

Find a mirror with plenty of light—the closer to daylight the better—and try to position yourself in front of the mirror in such a way that the light is evenly diffused over your face, with as few shadows as possible. You want to be able to see clearly enough so that you can easily spot areas where makeup may need more blending or smoothing, particularly around the cheeks or jaw line.

Cheeks

As you've already learned, the *Palmer Code* reveals that the cheek area is the most important component of facial beauty. Do you remember from Chapter Four how to use the imaginary grid to find the ideal shape of the cheeks? They should begin at the intersection that runs horizontally from the nostril and vertically down from the mid-pupillary line and of course, they should be round and full. If your cheeks do not follow this pattern, you can use makeup to mimic the ideal by creating the *illusion* of full cheeks in the perfect location.

Darker blush colors define the rounded portions and the inward contours of the cheeks, while lighter colors raise the cheeks from the face. This gives a fuller, more feminine shape.

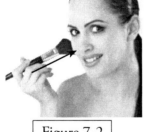

Figure 7-2

First, look for that ideal intersection on your face. Then form your ideal cheeks by highlighting the top using either a face highlighter or light-colored blush. At the bottom of the newly formed cheekbones, apply a darker blush from the imaginary gridline out toward the ear (see arrow fig 7-2). Use longer strokes of light color, continuing to apply until the color is just beginning to show, creating the illusion of a larger, fuller cheek.

Be sure to add a little color at a time and blend well. You want the blush to be dark enough to form the intended contours without creating any harsh lines. Once your blush is in place, you can use an extra-large makeup brush to smooth and blend the color (figure 7-2).

Remember, ideal cheeks are worth 75% of your *face number,* so spend as much time as it takes to master this one area. The improvement in your appearance and your *face number* make it well worth the time and effort.

> **Please remember this: you should strive to make the cheeks as close to ideal as you can make them, before looking to improve anything else.**

Eyes and Eyebrows

Eyebrows and eyes are the second most important elements of the *Palmer Code*, capturing attention and drawing people in as they talk to you. Figure 7-3 shows a perfectly shaped female eyebrow.

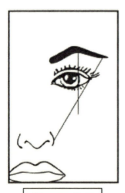

Figure 7-3

If your eyebrows are too bushy or form a less-than-ideal shape, you can use this illustration as your guide to sculpt them. A salon professional can create this shape by waxing, plucking, or threading, or you can pluck your eyebrows yourself. If you go to a professional, be very clear about what you're looking for as some salons follow varying patterns by default, such as round arches that are not an optimum aesthetic for your brows. You may want to bring this illustration as an example so that you are certain to capture the ideal shape. Remember the brow should begin in a club shape in alignment with the inside corner of the eye, angling to a high point that falls just outside the iris (colored portion of the eye). From there, the brow thins and tapers, ending on an imaginary diagonal from the outer nostril to the outside corner of the eye.

If your eyebrows are too low, too thin, or incomplete (eyebrows that lack the proper taper at the ends), use makeup to fill them in. You can use eye shadow for very light fill-in, but if you need more substantial lines use an eyebrow pencil. Either way, use a color that exactly matches your brow color. Feather in to cover sparse patches using short, light strokes, avoiding harsh lines (figure 7-4).

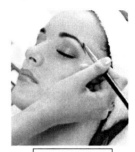

Figure 7-4

For low eyebrows, use an eyebrow pencil above the existing eyebrow to give the illusion of a brow that sits higher. If the eyebrow is incomplete, simply use the eyebrow pencil to complete the proper shape and taper.

After you have improved the eyebrow shape, it's time to accentuate the eyes. Depending on your age or your goal, taking care with eye makeup can help you brighten, widen, or actually give yourself an instant eye lift. Take a moment to review your eye score from "Chapter 5: Your Own Face Number and the Big Three". Look at your eyes and determine what you can do to most improve their appearance. Having a clear goal will help you focus your attention.

Eyeliner widens the eyes if you apply it just at the outer corners, about a quarter the way from corner toward center. Be careful to examine the look on your own eyes, as for some it can create a cross-eyed appearance. The more eyeliner you use, the smaller your eyes look.

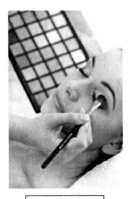

Figure 7-5

Eye shadow in the lid creases will de-emphasize dark circles, depressions or hollows, and excess skin or fatty tissue while accentuating the color and shape of your eyes. Brushes with shorter, stiffer bristles are useful when creating definition along the lash line, and longer bristles are ideal for allover application. For a natural look, use hues that match your skin tone, applying lighter colors on the lid and brow bone, and darker colors in the crease. Or, you can create a more dramatic look that widens the eyes by applying a darker color along the top lash line. After you've applied your color, switch to a large, soft eye shadow brush to blend well (figure 7-5).

You can also lengthen, curl, and thicken the eyelashes as another way of accentuating your eyes. False eyelashes, mascara, lash curlers, and even eyelash extensions from your salon are all tools you can use to create beautiful lashes. Just remember to confine the more dramatic of these to lowlight hours such as evening. Tools such as false eyelashes can look obvious in bright light.

The eyebrows and eyes can add up to 10 points to your *face number*, so spend a little time creating a great everyday look. You can have fun varying your look by using different colored shadows or even colored eye contacts, but you should establish a clear, natural-looking baseline for your day-to-day appearance. Once you've done that, you'll find it's quick and easy to maintain.

Lips

If you have beautiful lips, flaunt them! The mouth gives you a sensuous appearance, and a bright smile can light up a room. A simple sheer gloss can highlight already gorgeous lips.

If your lips are less than ideal, don't worry. They're probably the easiest features to shape using makeup. Lip liner (figure 7-6) can accentuate the lips vermillion borders and the cupid's bow (center upper lip V shape). Muted colors make the lips appear smaller while brighter reds and darker taupes create an illusion of fullness. Use your *Palmer Code* analysis from "Chapter 5: Your Own Face Number and the Big Three" to determine how to most effectively improve your lips. Once you have an idea of how your lips compare to the ideal, you can determine the best color tone to either soften or accentuate the size of the lips.

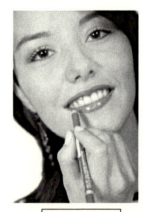

Figure 7-6

You should choose lip colors that borrow from your natural skin tones. The most important factor is to first determine what you'll use for everyday wear. Take a look at your natural lip color and then imagine how that color would look if you deepened the hue. That's your basis for choosing an everyday lip liner. Note that the color you choose may be very similar to your blush color. If that's the case, good: you are getting the feel for how to borrow from your natural flesh tones to choose colors that shape your beauty without drawing attention to the makeup itself. Once you have a naturally-toned lip liner, you can choose lipsticks with a bit more flexibility in palate (figure 7-7). It's a good idea to have a natural tone for everyday wear in lipsticks, but you can also play around with more color varieties to match clothing or express individual style.

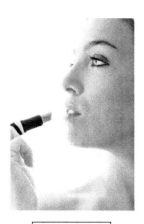

Figure 7-7

The *Palmer Code* states that the ratio of size to one another is the most important aspect of the lips. The ideal 3:4 ratio means that your upper lip should be about 75% as full and plump as the lower lip, giving the mouth a pleasing pout. How do your lips compare? If they fall short of the 3:4 ratio, you can use lip liner as an effective tool to sculpt your lips toward the ideal. For example, if your upper and lower lips are about the same size, you'll want to increase the size of your lower lip to create the illusion of the 3:4 ratio. To do this, simply fill in your lower lip with lip liner just along and *below* the lower edge.

Use the same trick on the top part if your upper lip is particularly thin. Run the lip liner just above the upper lip line, taking care to properly accentuate cupid's bow in order to create a fuller upper lip.

Regardless of how you've lined your lips to bring them closer to the 3:4 ratio, fill in the rest of the lips with the same lip liner to even out the look and create a solid base. You'll maintain color for a longer period of time. Lip liner can be your best friend.

The Palmer Code [Francis Palmer MD]

After your lip liner is in place, you can top it with a little lipstick if you'd like to vary the color, or for most situations, use a simple lip gloss. Almost everyone benefits from a little more softness and fullness overall, so consider using a sheer, satiny lip gloss during the day or a shiny gloss for nighttime drama.

Lips contribute 7% towards your *face number* and can have the hidden benefit of drawing in the observer's eye, thus diverting attention away from other facial features that are more difficult to shape using simple makeup tricks. In other words, it's easy to create perfect lips, so reap the rewards!

The Nose and the Rest of Your Face

In most cases, the nose benefits most when you divert focus away from it. If you've taken care with your cheeks, eyes, brows, and lips, you've already taken the biggest steps toward accomplishing that goal. Drawing focus toward your best features is the most effective way to de-emphasize the facial features that aren't so beneficial.

However, you can boost your beauty by using the same blush combinations you used on your face to shape your nose toward the ideal. To do this, first take a look at your analysis from "Chapter 6: Your Own Face Number for the Rest". In what ways, if any, did your nose fall short of the ideal? You may have found that your nose may be on the broad side, or perhaps it's long and narrow. If there are any "off" features, you can easily camouflage them using blush.

If you have a wide nose, you can bring your nose back to proportion using shading and highlights. Run a thin line of highlight along your nose from top to tip (figure 7-8). Then, use your blush brush (figure 7-9) to shade along the sides of the tip with darker colors. You can pinch the bristles between your thumb and forefinger to maintain better control on the brush and therefore create more distinct contours. Highlighting the sides with darker shading causes your nose to appear more slim and sleek. You can use the same technique to hide any irregularities. Darker colors hide and de-emphasize bumps while lighter colors fill in depressions or grooves. The end result should always be a slim, sleek, unobserved nose.

Narrow the nose with dark colors on the sides.

Lighter colors across the top make the nose appear slimmer.

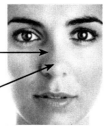

Figure 7-8

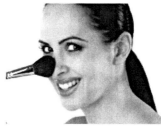

Figure 7-9

Use these same techniques to highlight the jaw line, chin and neck areas (figure 7-10).

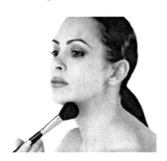

Figure 7-10

Finally, use the proper color foundation to de-emphasize uneven areas of skin pigmentation, loose skin and wrinkling.

I think it's also worth mentioning permanent makeup. If you have little or no eyebrows, you might want to consider having them permanently placed using eyebrow tattooing. In the right situation and when performed to create the proper shape as described numerous times in this book, tattooing eyebrows is a very real and effective method of getting great looking eyebrows. Make sure your technician is experienced and understands what you want. Cosmetic tattooing is a permanent procedure and it's important to feel confident that the technician knows what to do and understands the proper facial aesthetics to give you great looking eyebrows. The same can be said for permanent eyeliner and lip liner. When properly done, these can add real aesthetic improvement to the eyes and lips.

The Palmer Code [Francis Palmer MD]

Your Hair

Your hair can frame your face in ways that can actually boost your *face number.* For men, facial hair can camouflage imperfections while adding strong angles to create the chiseled structure so desirable in the male face. Hairstyles are similar to makeup in that the end goal is to accentuate your facial features.

If you have ideal or very close to ideal "big three" facial features, by all means show them off. You can wear your hair long, short, or off of your face and any one of these styles will complement your great facial features. If however, your facial features are less than ideal it's not a good idea to let them out there by themselves or you will appear less attractive (lower *face number*). Instead you'll want to wear hairstyles that frame the face, adding emphasis to the cheeks.

The following maneuver will illustrated this point. Look straight into a mirror and pull all of the hair away from your face. Does your face look soft and feminine or does it appear more angular? If it's looking angular, position your hands palms-down and cup your ears. You'll see this adds volume to the face and makes it appear more soft and feminine. That's the type of hairstyle that will soften a female face that has relatively flat cheeks.

Bangs are an excellent solution for many facial imperfections. Consider wearing bangs if you have any of these:

- High forehead
- Less-than-ideal eyebrows
- Full eyelids
- Wrinkled forehead

Bangs will deemphasize all of the above while framing your eyes and cheeks.

Men, you want a face that appears angular, rugged and masculine, so select a hairstyle that emphasizes a chiseled facial structure and avoid those that soften your features. Short hair with strong, angled lines tend to look best for men. Longer hair, especially if loose in front of the ears, can soften the male face causing the *face number* to decrease.

Exercise is an Important Key to Your Face Number

You might be surprised to learn that you can increase your *face number* by changing one single element of your daily routine: exercise your face. You exercise your body, why not your face? Your face has muscles that need exercise to remain firm and toned. Toned muscles increase the elasticity and firmness of facial skin. In other words, the skin and tissues of your face resist sagging. I'm going to share some excellent facial exercises on the next few pages, however as with any exercise, you should consult your doctor before trying them.

We all understand that if we don't exercise our muscles they'll eventually become weak. When you have a cast your broken arm or leg, what happens? Because you can't exercise those muscles, they weaken (atrophy) and your arm or leg looks smaller when the cast is finally removed. This illustrates the fact that our muscles, including those of the face, get smaller and weaker if we don't exercise them. The good news is, *that five minutes a day is all it takes to strengthen these muscles for improved facial shape and tone.* Ideally, you would begin using these exercises in your twenties to maintain a youthful, toned face and neck. But you can reap the benefits by starting these simple exercises at any age and obtain a noticeable improvement. I do mine in the car every day as I drive to work. It's easy, fast and highly effective.

Cheek muscles

Figure 7-11 shows the facial muscles, including the ones that you can strengthen in order to improve your *face number*. By now, I hope you can guess which facial muscles are the most important to your *face number*. That's right: the ones that affect the cheeks.

Arrows depict the location of the cheek muscles that can pull the soft tissues back onto the cheeks when properly exercised.

Exaggerated smiling can be used to strengthen the cheek muscles by contracting the muscles that push the tissue of the face upward and outwards towards the ear. This translates to a more youthful cheek shape which could have a significant impact on your *face number*.

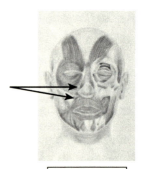

Figure 7-11

When you first try this, or any of the exercises described in this book, do them gently until you become accustomed to their effects. Perform the smile exercise (figure 7-12) by opening your mouth and exaggerating your smile, to its fullest extent, while slowly counting to 10. Once you reach 10, relax for a few seconds and then repeat the process again 10 times. Think of this as doing reps (repetitions) just like when you're in the gym working out your biceps or triceps. As you do this exercise, you'll feel your muscles tighten and the next day your cheeks might actually be sore, just like other muscles after a good workout. It only takes a few minutes, requires no special equipment, no gym membership, no personal trainer and you can even do them in the shower or while driving to and from work, as I do.

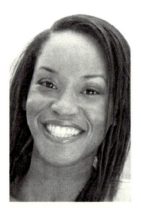

Figure 7-12

Using this technique every day will not only firm and tone muscles, preventing them from premature sagging, it could also help maintain the elasticity and tone of your facial skin.

Eye Area (Eye and Eyebrow) Muscles

You can exercise your eyebrows and eyes using a similar technique. Looking at the face muscles (figure 7-13), we see that the forehead has large muscles that, when contracted, lift and elevate the tissues of the forehead

[Francis Palmer MD] The Palmer Code

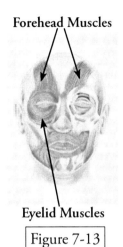

Forehead Muscles

Eyelid Muscles

Figure 7-13

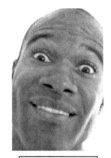

Figure 7-14

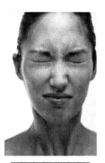

Figure 7-15

including the eyebrows. To do this exercise, simply lift the forehead and eyebrows using an inquisitive expression (figure 7-14). Do similar reps as suggested for the cheek exercises. Daily exercise of this sort can raise the eyebrows and or prevent them from falling to a less ideal position.

The eyelid muscles, which are seen as circular muscles surrounding the eyes (figure 7-13), can be exercised by forcibly squinting (figure 7-15). This contracts the eye muscles, strengthening them to resist gravity and the aging process. Do these in reps of 10, similar to what you do for the cheeks and forehead muscles. One thing to note, however, is that it's possible these exercises may increase facial wrinkling but any resultant wrinkling should be minor and far outweighed by the beneficial contouring and toning results these exercises may provide.

Toning the neck

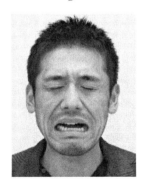

Figure 7-16

To strengthen and tone the neck, open and curve down the corners of your mouth while moving the lower jaw slightly forward (figure 7-16). This causes the muscles of the neck to contract. This maneuver takes a little time to master but is well worth the effort. If you want to maintain a smooth, tight neck do this exercise daily but do not clench your teeth while performing this maneuver as this may damage your teeth or temperomandibular joint.

The Palmer Code   [Francis Palmer MD]

Visit our website www.whatsyournumbernews.com to view a video demonstration of these and other exercises. So many reasons to do these simple exercises...and all of them can increase your *face number*. Try it today and do it for life.

Skin Care and the Palmer Code

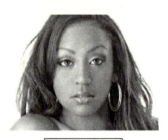

Figure 7-17

Beautiful skin can increase your *face number*. If you are in your teens, you should think about maintaining your skin by avoiding sun damage and using a simple skin maintenance program. This means daily use of a good UVA/UVB sunscreen of SPF 30 or greater (SPF 30 blocks out ~ 97 % of harmful UV rays while an SPF 45 may only add an additional 2-3% blockage... but at triple the cost). Repeating the application of an SPF 30 sunscreen every 2-3 hours is much more effective, at reducing UV exposure, than a single application of an SPF 45.

As you enter your twenties, thirties and beyond, it's better to embrace a long-term, goal-oriented approach to your skin. Think of adding periodic facials and skin rejuvenating products that promote collagen formation in the skin.

With so many skin care products on the market today, how are you supposed to know what's right for you? I advise you to keep it simple. Your goal should be skin that is toned and soft, like a baby's skin. To achieve this, look for products that build collagen, moisturize and block the sun.

Youthful, healthy, beautiful skin has collagen, lots and lots of collagen. The problem is, as we age and are exposed to UV rays from the sun, our collagen is damaged and depleted. This leads to skin that appears dull, rough, lined, wrinkled and loose.

The illustration (figure 7-18), shows a cross-section of the skin. Beneath the outer layer

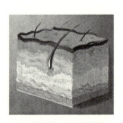

Figure 7-18

(epidermis) lies the dermis where dense collagen makes the baby's skin appear smooth, soft, plump and beautiful. As this collagen layer is depleted with age, sun exposure or harsh chemicals, the skin appears rough, loose and wrinkled. So how can you maintain or increase the amount of collagen in your skin? We'll save that discussion until later in this chapter but let's first look at how you can keep the collagen you have. To maintain collagen, follow these simple steps:

1. **Avoid overexposure to the sun or damaging UV rays from tanning booths.**

2. **Hydrate the skin.**

Healthy skin must have the proper amount of moisture. This simple, skin-saving fact is often overlooked or misunderstood. The following analogy demonstrates the importance of hydration to healthy beautiful looking skin. You see two leaves on the ground. One leaf is green and moist while the other is brown, dry and brittle. Now ask yourself, which one has more lines and wrinkles? The answer, the dry one of course. Your skin is no different. Drink plenty of water every day, avoid skin products containing harsh chemicals that can strip the oils and moisture from your skin and use a daily moisturizer to maintain proper hydration.

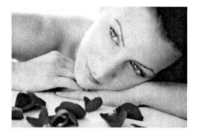

Figure 7-19

3. **You are what you eat...and this is reflected by your skin.**

Avoid junk and fast foods. Instead, eat a healthy diet rich in fruits and vegetables that rank high in the ORAC (Oxygen Radical Absorbance Capacity) scale. Foods like wolfberries, prunes, blueberries, garlic, spinach and others contain anti-oxidant capabilities that may help maintain your skin.

The Palmer Code [Francis Palmer MD]

Finally, here are some helpful tips regarding your skin and the sun. If you crave the tanned look, use self tanners, but stay away from excessive sun exposure (and yes, that includes the tanning booths). Excess UV exposure is the number one cause of premature aging of your skin. Always be aware of your environment because the amount of UV exposure you receive increases by 10% for every 1,000 feet you rise in elevation. Even when sitting in the shade, you may get as much as 70% or more UV exposure as you get from direct sunlight. UV rays are reflected off water, sand, concrete and snow surfaces, increasing the amount of UV exposure. Even on a cloudy day, you could get 80% of the UV rays from a sunny day.

Now that you know how to protect and maintain your skin's collagen, let's look at the ways of increasing the collagen in your skin. Beautiful, healthy, youthful looking skin doesn't just happen...you must have a plan. Follow this simple 3-step process for beautiful skin.

Skin Care Steps

Step One: Prepare the skin

This seems like such a simple step and yet it's overlooked by many people because they simply don't understand just how important this is to an effective overall skin program. In this step a gentle cleanser removes the surface oils from the skin. Unlike soaps that may remove oils but leave a filmy residue, a gentle cleanser allows other skin rejuvenating products to penetrate the skin layers where they'll be more effective. Preparing the skin means different things depending on the type of skin you have. As we just mentioned, cleansers remove surface oils from the skin. Refining grains, containing small abrasive beads, allow for gentle exfoliation of the outer skin layers. (These layers become thickened with age and sun exposure, creating a barrier that prevents skin rejuvenating products from penetrating into the deeper layers). Toners using an astringent, like alpha hydroxy acid, will remove debris from pores allowing them to appear less prominent. Depending on your skin type (dry, normal,

[Francis Palmer MD] The Palmer Code

oily or a mixture), you'll prepare the skin by using one or more of these product types. Once you've prepared the skin, the tissue is ready to accept the full benefits of skin rejuvenating products.

Step Two: Rejuvenate the skin.

Smooth, soft, beautiful skin has collagen, and lots of it. Rejuvenation of the skin is accomplished by replacing depleted collagen and promoting increased hydration within the skin layers. There are many types of skin rejuvenating products that can accomplish this goal. Skin care ingredients like Vitamin A, C, and E have been around for years. Newcomers like DMAE, DHAE, alpha lipoic acid, Co-Q10, copper peptides, hyaluronic acid, N6-Furfurladenine (Kinerase), retinyl palmitate, penta/hexa and neuro-peptides are all the latest rage. All of these ingredients act in a slightly different manner but they are generally regarded as effective skin rejuvenating agents. It's also important to understand that no matter the key ingredient, effective products must contain adequate concentrations of that key ingredient, so be sure to read the label to see what's in the creams you're buying and using.

You may wish to use two or three products that work together to accelerate the rejuvenation process. I like to think of this as "cross training for the skin". For example, you may use a product containing Kinerase as the active rejuvenating agent for 2 weeks, then rotate a different product based on pentapeptides for 2 weeks, and finally, complete the cycle with a product containing Co-Q10. Continue by repeating the cycle. For more advanced skin rejuvenation, consider using two or more similar products simultaneously, The result is a synergistic and accumulative effect.

Step Three: Protect the skin.

Protection begins with daily use of a good sunscreen, and avoidance of excess sun exposure. Sorry, I'll say it again, suntan booths are a big no-no. Proper nutrition and hydration should also be a part of your daily routine.

The Palmer Code [Francis Palmer MD]

In addition to your daily cleanser and daily skin rejuvenating cream, you should also use a gentle exfoliating agent once a week. Once you're in your forties and beyond, also consider additional skin rejuvenating creams that further smooth the skin and soften unwanted lines, wrinkles (using some of the ingredients mentioned in Step Two above) and areas of uneven pigmentation (using ingredients like hydroquinone, kojic acid, licorice.)

In addition to the three steps of basic skin care, you may choose to consider medical skin procedures. These include mild chemical peels, microdermabrasion, radiofrequency, superficial Laser and IPL (Intense Pulsed Light) treatments. These typically involve a series of treatments in the office (or medi-spa), with minimal down time. Discuss these treatments with your doctor if you feel your skin requires extra care and seek out an experienced professional that you can trust.

Weight Gain and Loss to Shape the face

The fatty tissues in your face contribute to facial shape. The proper amount will make the face appear healthy and aesthetically balanced but if you're seeking to alter your body fat, you should understand that weight loss also decreases the amount of fat in the face. In extreme cases of weight loss, this can and does lead to increased facial angularity. For women this may make the face appear elongated and relatively masculine, which will decrease your *face number*. The converse is also true. Weight gain will plump out the neck, cheeks and nasolabial folds. In women over the age of thirty, it's advantageous to maintain a body weight that supports the proper amount of facial fat, enabling the face to appear soft and feminine while focusing on shaping the body with Pilates or yoga.

Beautiful Teeth Enhance Your Smile

Your lips are aesthetically important to an attractive mouth, but so is a beautiful smile. Smiling has been shown to elicit positive emotions in not only the person smiling, but in those observing the smile.

Part of a beautiful smile is aesthetically pleasing teeth. Caps, veneers and teeth whitening are all ways to create that perfect smile. Dentures, bridges and even teeth implants are becoming more popular. Of course, you should strive to maintain proper and consistent dental hygiene to maintain your teeth. Fresh breath and properly aligned white teeth all contribute to a pleasing appearance.

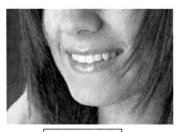

Figure 7-20

A Full, Thick Head of Hair

It'll come as no surprise that both men and women get a boost from a full head of hair. Good nutrition can help promote soft, beautiful hair, as can supplements that include omega 3 fatty acids in the form of fish oils and other oils.

For pattern baldness, there are medications available that are designed to slow down or reverse hair loss. Rogaine and Propecia are the most common. They do require topical scalp application or that you take a pill everyday for life. Alternatively, one can use wigs, hair weaves, or toupees as non-medical ways of camouflaging the hair loss. Just bear in mind that nowadays, a man's fully bald head has come into style. A shaved head accentuates strong male features, and can be quite attractive. Experiment with a look that's right for you.

Now that you have learned your *face number* and how to improve it, let's move on to the next chapter and explore your *body number* within the *Palmer Code*.

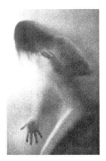

Chapter 8: The Palmer Code Body

It has been said that the body "is a temple," and your body is obviously important, so let's look at how different factors like body size, shape, and proportion affect the *outer you* and *your number.*

As with the face, the *Palmer Code* reveals the secrets of specific, ideal patterns as they relate to the body's external beauty. By learning how to identify these patterns, you can control your body's aesthetics to a far greater extent than you might have previously imagined. We'll get into how that works in the next chapters, but for now, let's look at the ideal and how it relates to your body.

You'll want to use a clear, objective eye as you take a look at your body in this initial self-evaluation. Keep in mind that your body is very personal, and for some, this exercise may cause some anxiety, but I challenge you to set all that aside during the self-analysis process. In fact I'll go so far as to prescribe, as your beauty doctor, that you eliminate self-critical emotions and judgments *forever* when it comes to your image. If you want to improve your look and take your body to its ultimate state—for both inner and outer beauty—getting emotional and judgmental will never help. While evaluation is all about finding the facts, being judgmental is self-limiting because our objectivity becomes clouded by prejudice and emotions. For those reasons being objective is helpful, but being judgmental is not.

The Palmer Code   [Francis Palmer MD]

Your best approach is to follow the very same strategy I outlined for you right from the beginning. The same strategy that you can use to improve and beautify any aspect of your life:

1. Define specific key elements
2. Evaluate yourself
3. Focus on what's important

Remember using this three-stage approach when you conceived your gorgeous imaginary garden in the beginning of the book? Well, you can use the same process to realize your ideal body; and you can do it with delight, respect and love for yourself making every step an enjoyable and enlightening experience.

If you feel any anxiety at all in relation to the body evaluation, you may wish to jump ahead and read Chapters 13 and 14 that deal with the *inner you*. There you will learn, among other things, how to control your emotions, your environment and how you can harness the hidden beauty potential and power stored within you. Consider this your first *inner you* challenge: self-analysis of your body is causing a stress response message. Are you going to sound the alarm and kick your sympathetic nervous system and hormones into high gear and run away? Or, are you going to override that stressed out emotion with relaxation messages that keep anxiety, fear, and high blood pressure at bay? That's just one of the coping mechanism you'll learn in Chapter 14, "Unlocking the Inner You". You can make a conscious decision to diffuse stress and enter that optimum realm where you learn how to flourish and grow.

If you need to take a moment, by all means please do so. You may want to try the following relaxation exercise. Close your eyes, relax, and focus on your breathing. Ten slow deep breaths should do it. Then take an imaginary journey someplace that delights you. Perhaps you'll want to go for a walk in your garden. Personally, I like to imagine myself at the beach. I find that the more detail I am able to visualize in my mind's eye—the sound of the waves, the feel of the sun and sea breeze, the smell of the saltwater and the sparkling scenery—the deeper my state of relaxation. Look for these types of details in your imaginary place, and just hang out there for a little while. When you feel you're fully relaxed and ready to come back, count your breaths backwards from ten down to one.

When you're ready, we'll get started.

Body Evaluation

There are numerous aspects of body form that contribute to *your number*. These are listed below (table 8-1) along with point values for the *Palmer Code* body:

POINT SYSTEM FOR THE PALMER CODE BODY			
WOMEN		**MEN**	
Upper-to-lower body ratio	30 points	Upper-to-lower body ratio	25 points
Hips and legs	20 points	Shoulders	18 points
Breasts	18 points	Chest	15 points
Buttocks	17 points	Abdomen	12 points
Abdomen and waist	10 points	Arms	10 points
Shoulders and arms	3 points	Buttocks	8 points
Skin	2 points	Hips and waist	7 points
Total	**100 points**	Legs	4 points
		Skin	1 point
		Total	**100 points**

Table 8-1

Upper-to-Lower Body Ratio

Think of someone who has a sexy body. Now think about what makes that person sexy.

When you think about "what's hot" among the sexes, the upper-to-lower body ratio may not be the first thing that comes to mind.

The Palmer Code [Francis Palmer MD]

However, this is the single most important aspect of body aesthetics. It's one of those things that just "looks right" to the human eye, even if you don't realize what it's about or why the individual appears attractive.

So what is it, exactly?

The upper-to-lower body ratio is the length of the upper body compared to the lower body or simply stated, how much of your body's height is comprised by your legs. For example, if you have a 35/65 upper-to-lower body ratio your upper body is 35% of your overall height while your lower body makes up the remaining 65% and you appear to have long legs (figure 8-2). This ratio is a good indication of how balanced your body appears. When this ratio is off the body appears top or bottom-heavy and as a result, out of balance.

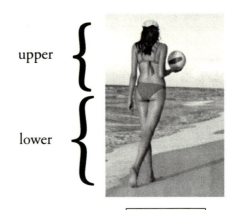

Figure 8-2

For women, the ideal ratio is 40/60 to 35/65, which reflects a body with longer legs. Do you remember the discussion at the beginning of this book about Phi and the golden ratio? Coincidentally, a woman's ideal upper-to-lower body ratio falls within the vicinity of the Phi formula.

For men, the ideal is closer to an even balanced 45/55 to 50/50.

You can determine your upper-to-lower body ratio by measuring and working out exact percentages, but you certainly can "eyeball it." Stand in front of a full-length mirror. Anything above the narrowest part of your waist is your upper body; anything below that is your lower body. Determine the length proportion of upper to lower. Following are some examples to help you along.

[Francis Palmer MD] The Palmer Code

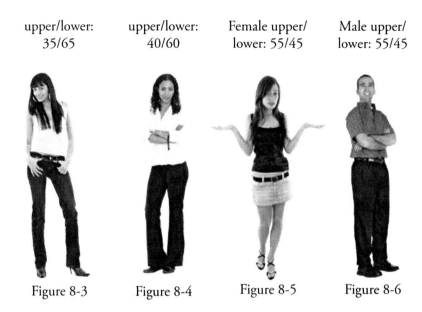

Figure 8-3 — upper/lower: 35/65
Figure 8-4 — upper/lower: 40/60
Figure 8-5 — Female upper/lower: 55/45
Figure 8-6 — Male upper/lower: 55/45

Assign yourself points using figures 8-3 to 8-6 for your upper-to-lower body ratio according to the following scale (table 8-2):

Points

Upper-to-Lower Body Ratio
Up to 30 points for women
Up to 25 points for men

	WOMEN		MEN	
	35/65	30 points	45/55	25 points
	40/60	30 points	50/50	25 points
	45/55	25 points	40/60	20 points
	50/50	20 points	55/45	15 points
	60/40	15 points	60/40	10 points
	70/30	10 points	70/30	5 points

Table 8-2

The Palmer Code   [Francis Palmer MD]

Hips

For women, this feature is aesthetically linked to the legs. Ideally female hips are trim but curvaceous with legs that are long, lean, toned, and smooth. This accounts for a possible 20 points for women. Compare yourself to figures 8-7 to 8-10.

Points

Hips and Legs
Up to 20 points for women

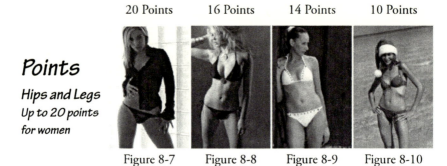

20 Points — Figure 8-7
16 Points — Figure 8-8
14 Points — Figure 8-9
10 Points — Figure 8-10

For men, hips are less aesthetically important and account for 7 points in the *Palmer Code*. The ideal male hips are thin, flat and square which accentuates the shoulders, a key beauty element for men (see figures 8-11 to 8-13 opposite page).

[Francis Palmer MD] The Palmer Code

Points

Hips
Up to 7 points for men

7 Points   5 Points   3 Points

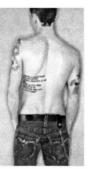 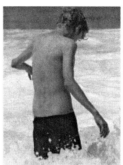

Figure 8-11   Figure 8-12   Figure 8-13

Ideally, male legs are the epitome of power, speed and strength. Well-defined, muscular legs are worth a possible 4 points total (figures 8-14 and 8-15).

Legs (Men)

Points

Legs
Up to 4 points for men

4 Points   3 Points

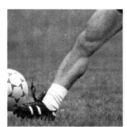 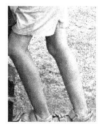

Figure 8-14   Figure 8-15

The Palmer Code [Francis Palmer MD]

Chest

The female breast is a thing of beauty with soft, gentle yet flowing contours. Size is less relevant within the *Palmer Code* than overall breast shape. Ideal breasts are upturned with more fullness in the lower portion giving it a soft, sloping curvature and tear-drop shape. The breasts should be relatively symmetric in size and position on the chest, with areolae that are not too large or small when compared to the overall breast. For women, breasts contribute a maximum of 18 points to the *Palmer Code* calculation for the body (figures 8-16 through 8-21).

Points

Breasts
Up to 18 points for women

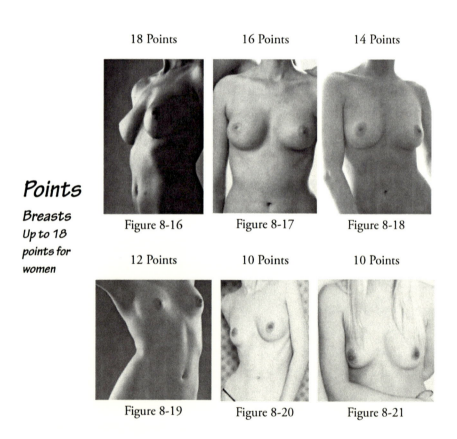

18 Points — Figure 8-16
16 Points — Figure 8-17
14 Points — Figure 8-18
12 Points — Figure 8-19
10 Points — Figure 8-20
10 Points — Figure 8-21

For men the ideal chest is thick, muscular, well-defined and is worth 15 total possible points. The pectoralis muscle shapes the contours and, along with strong shoulders, creates the ideal V-shaped torso (see figures 8-22 to 8-25 below).

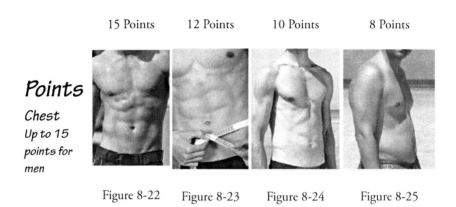

Points

Chest
Up to 15 points for men

Figure 8-22   Figure 8-23   Figure 8-24   Figure 8-25

Buttocks

For both men and women, the ideal buttocks should be full, round and toned. Buttocks contribute 17 total possible points for women (figure 8-26 to 8-28) and 8 total possible points for men (figures 8-29 to 8-31).

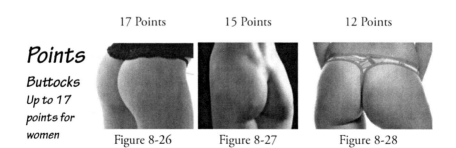

Points

Buttocks
Up to 17 points for women

Figure 8-26   Figure 8-27   Figure 8-28

The Palmer Code [Francis Palmer MD]

Points
Buttocks
Up to 8 points for men

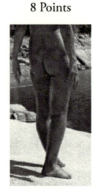
8 Points
Figure 8-29

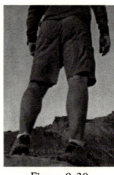
6 Points
Figure 8-30

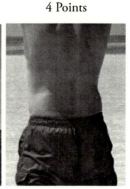
4 Points
Figure 8-31

Abdomen

There's little doubt that great-looking abs enhance a beautiful body for both men and women. Ideally, the abdomen is flat and toned. Women look best with a small waist in proportion to the hips—creating the ideal hourglass shape.

Men ideally have visible muscular definition; hard cut, or the proverbial six-pack abs. The abdomen and waist together contribute 10 possible points for women (figure 8-32 to 8-34) and up to 12 points for men (figure 8-35 to 8-37).

Points
Abs & Waist
Up to 10 points for women

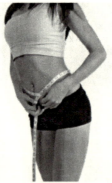
10 Points
Figure 8-32

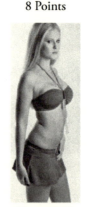
8 Points
Figure 8-33

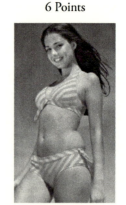
6 Points
Figure 8-34

[Francis Palmer MD] The Palmer Code

Points

Abs

Up to 12 points for men

12 Points 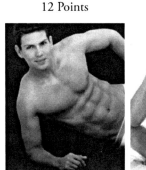 10 Points 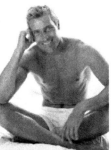 6 Points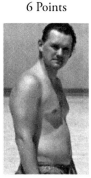

Figure 8-35   Figure 8-36   Figure 8-37

Shoulders and Arms

For women, the shoulders and arms should be toned and firm, contributing 3 points to the *Palmer Code*. Unless the shoulders and arms are noticeably heavy or thin, simply give yourself 3 points.

Points

Shoulders & Arms

Up to 3 points for women

3 Points

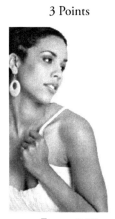

Figure 8-38

In men, these areas play a more significant role in the *Palmer Code* for the body. Men's shoulders should be broad, toned with well-developed muscles. The arms should be toned and muscular, thereby completing the upper body package with a show of strength and power.

The Palmer Code [Francis Palmer MD]

For men, shoulders are worth 18 points and the arms are worth 10 points (see figure 8-39 to 8-44 below).

Points
Shoulders
Up to 18 points for men

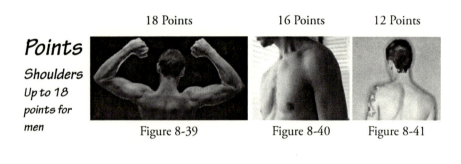

18 Points — Figure 8-39
16 Points — Figure 8-40
12 Points — Figure 8-41

Points
Arms
Up to 10 points for men

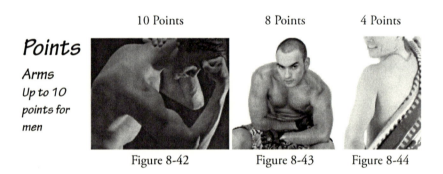

10 Points — Figure 8-42
8 Points — Figure 8-43
4 Points — Figure 8-44

Skin

Skin of the body is worth 2 points for women and 1 point for men. In either case, skin looks best when it's toned, smooth, and firm. If your skin is free of blemishes or irregularities in pigment or laxity, give yourself the full point value according to your gender.

2 Points

Points
Skin
Up to 2 points for women
Up to 1 point for men

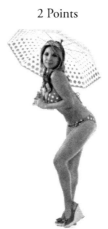

Figure 8-45

Your Body Prescription

During the course of this chapter, you may have discovered that you've been overly critical of yourself in the past when it comes to how you view your body or conversely, you may have zeroed in on some key areas you'd like to improve. Either way, I hope you've learned something new, because that's what the self-development process is all about.

The next step is to take those areas of focus and develop a strategy for realizing your best self. As you begin, be mindful of which specific areas you want to enhance. Focusing your attention in this manner allows you to set priorities based on their aesthetic importance to your *body number*. To help you along, you may want to refer back to the point system for the *Palmer Code* Body in the table at the beginning of this chapter.

The next two chapters will help you learn how to unlock your body's full potential. This is exciting for me, because I want you to look your best—your absolute, fantasy ideal—with as little effort as possible. For example, I often see patients who, despite working hard at the gym or paying for expensive personal trainers, are disappointed

The Palmer Code [Francis Palmer MD]

with their results. I believe this happens when you don't have a clear vision of what you are trying to achieve or don't completely understand the various ways that your body will respond to specific exercises. It frustrates me to see all that wasted time, money and effort.

I'll show you the full spectrum of how to take your body to its highest achievable level in my book, *"What's Your Number" The Palmer Code Ultimate Body*. In the meantime, let's look at how you can take control right now to create lasting and effective change.

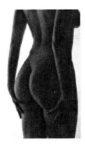

Chapter 9: Women, Unlock Your Palmer Code Body

At once long and lean yet soft and curvaceous, the female form is a work of living art, celebrated by painters and sculptors and artists of all stripes. Your shape might be square, round, rectangular, or the classic hourglass figure of legends like Sophia Loren and Marilyn Monroe.

No matter the starting point, you can regulate your weight and use the various secrets of the *Palmer Code* to improve upon your body in a precise and consistent manner, which means that you are in control. Once you consciously accept that fact, you might find that you have a lot more success (and a lot more peace of mind) in improving and fine-tuning what you already have.

In fact, as a modern woman, you have a lot of choices when it comes to shaping your body with fashion. With the right clothing, you can achieve an hourglass figure even if you're shaped more like a banana or an apple underneath your clothes. Let's break it down piece-by-piece.

Upper-to-Lower Body Ratio

We discussed the upper-to-lower body ratio and how it has the greatest impact on your *body number*. For women, you may recall the ideal is a 35/65 to 40/60 ratio, which accentuates the length of the legs. If your score fell short of the maximum 30 points, consider some of the following tactics to enhance your upper-to-lower body ratio and make your legs appear longer:

The Palmer Code [Francis Palmer MD]

High heels. I'm sure you're already familiar with them. They're not for everybody, but they're a quick fix to add more length to the leg. And for women, the upper-to-lower body ratio is essentially all about long legs.

Stretching exercises. Even if your legs aren't as long as you'd like them to be, you can create the illusion by lengthening the muscles. Yoga, Pilates, and other stretching exercises are a good way to achieve long, toned (as opposed to bulky) muscles. Thinner legs also add to this illusion. Just remember that bulk—regardless of whether it's coming from muscle or fat—will give the illusion of a shorter looking leg. Go for length.

Clothing. Choose clothing that makes your legs appear longer. High-waists, dark colors, slimming pants (stay away from pleats) are a good start. For even more length, consider a long, straight pant that finishes in a high heel of the same color.

Hips and Legs

As they say, nothing beats a great pair of legs, and as the second most relevant feature to the *Palmer Code* Body score, it seems that's the case. Shape, length, girth, and tone of the legs contribute to making your body beautiful.

In women, curved hips with the upper leg longer than the lower leg are considered ideal. The full, curvaceous female hip gives the body the lower portion of the hour-glass body shape. The calf should be shapely but not so large as to overshadow the long, lean overall appearance to the leg. The leg should look fit but not overly muscular, as too much muscle bulk makes the legs look relatively short and squat. Similarly, legs that are too thin look less attractive.

For great hips and legs, you can follow many of the same strategies for achieving the ideal upper-to-lower body ratio:

Stretching exercises. I can't say it enough. The ultimate goal here is to lengthen and tone, not build muscle bulk. Your goal is to achieve long, lean muscles in your legs. Yoga and Pilates help build these muscles in such a way that will result in shapely hips and legs. Beware of thigh-burning exercises or heavy weight-lifting that can create too much muscle bulk.

Aerobics. These exercises are basically anything that increases your heart rate. Aerobics are good exercises for the hips and legs because most muscle-targeted reps come in the form of resistance or calisthenics, not weight lifting and the focus is on toning.

Healthy eating. Too much weight on the legs can make them look shorter. If you're not at your ideal weight, make small changes in your daily intake (because drastic changes inevitably result in disappointment) until you're at the best weight for you.

Hemline. Most women look best in skirts or dress that fall right at the knee. The knee is the narrowest part of your leg, and clothing at that length gives the illusion of slimmer legs. It's OK to wear a hemline that is shorter or longer, just be mindful of where that line falls. If you have substantial calf muscles, a hemline that cuts across the widest part of your calf will give the illusion of stouter legs, so be careful.

Clothing cuts. If you want to give your hips a more slimming look, there are lots of clothing options that will help. Tops with a straight cut neckline across the collarbone balance the hips, as do a-line skirts. Also, wear pants cut in a straight line from waist to foot. Avoid tapered, boot cut, or pleated pants, as anything that adds curve to the line will add curves to your figure. Conversely, do wear these styles if you feel your hips could use a little more roundness and curve.

Breasts

Remember, when it comes to breasts, shape is more relevant to the *Palmer Code* than size.

In addition to the classic teardrop shape and upturned aereola, there's another important aspect of how your breasts contribute to your body's beauty and your *body number*. It turns out that the breasts provide balance to the hips, thereby contributing to an overall sense of body proportion.

Notice in figure 9-2, how the breasts are related to the hips. Roughly speaking, the female breast should approach a vertical line drawn up from the hips, as depicted in the image on the right. This is a general rule, however, not hard and fast, because the ideal female breast is more than this one aspect. Here are some ways to affect the shape and fullness of the breasts.

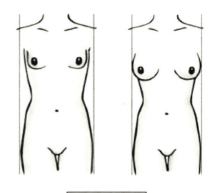

Figure 9-2

Body shapers. Look for bras that offer support and if possible, accentuate the balance portrayed in the illustration on the right in figure 9-2 above. Another option is to use gel inserts, padded bras, push-up bras and other items available to help you bring your shape toward the ideal.

Exercise. Obviously, there are no exercises that shape the breast itself, as breasts are not comprised of muscle tissue. However, exercising the underlying pectoralis muscle can give breasts a solid foundation, and can often help to achieve the desired upturned angle.

Posture. Do not slouch due to self-consciousness or for any other reason. Regardless of your breast size, shape, or positioning, your body beauty will benefit from sitting straight and standing straight.

Clothing. A good wardrobe stand-by is a v-necked button-down that opens to just where the contours begin. This helps to balance both the minimal and the ample bosom.

Buttocks

Toned, round, and firm is the ideal. Use these tips to improve the shape of your buttocks.

Nutrition and exercise. If you want to slim you buttocks, the most important step is to monitor your eating until you reach your ideal weight. During the process, turn to stretching exercises such as yoga and Pilates to firm and tone the underlying muscles. To add more shape to the buttocks, consider targeted muscle-building exercises that add bulk. At the gym, this means fewer repetitions at higher weights and slow, careful movements. Throughout the day, be sure to take the stairs instead of the elevator whenever possible and if you really want to work those glutes, go up the stairs backwards. Just be sure to use the handrail.

Clothing. Always be sure to check your backside when trying on clothes. A-line and pencil skirts tend to flatter any rear. When selecting jeans and pants, take careful note of how they fit. Make sure your clothes fit both the buttocks *and* the waist. Take note of the pockets and be sure they are positioned in a way that is flattering. Straight cuts in the back tend to have a flattening and slimming effect, whereas pockets add curve. Pockets can also camouflage, however, especially in jeans, so take a careful look and buy accordingly.

Abdomen

Rock hard abs, a lean core, and a thin waist are all the rage. If that sounds like you, congratulations! If not, you still have plenty of options.

Nutrition and exercise. Here again, there's no substitute or shortcut for reaching and maintaining your ideal weight. When it comes to exercise, focus on workouts that target your core. You can even focus on your core throughout your day by clenching your abs while sitting or walking.

Clothing. Belts can help accentuate the waist, and wider belts can help to camouflage a thick belly. Wear shirts and jackets that taper at the small of the back. And as always, avoid pleated pants.

Compression. Slimming clothing, girdles, and compression garments are available and are often quite effective. Just be mindful of the "muffin top" effect, defined as a softness at the waist when wearing tight jeans or girdles that end below the belly button. When in doubt, choose smooth lines over ones that cinch here and balloon out there.

The Palmer Code [Francis Palmer MD]

Shoulders and Arms

Female shoulders and arms look best when toned without appearing overly muscular. Like the nose on the face, the shoulders and arms should blend in with the rest of the body and not distract the observer's gaze.

Weight training. Lighter weights with more repetition is the key to muscle toning.

Stretching. Yoga, Pilates, and swimming are all excellent activities for toning and firming the shoulders and arms.

Skin

For women, body skin should be almost as smooth, supple, and consistent in complexion and pigmentation as that of the face. Take extra care with your skin because once damaged, it's more difficult to make it look youthful and refreshed.

Sun. It is so important to avoid excess sun exposure. UV rays—regardless of whether they are from the sun or the tanning bed—can cause premature aging and result in lax, wrinkled and rough skin. Limit your UV exposure and opt for self tanners instead. If you must be in the sun, be sure to use a high quality sun screen with both UVA and UVB protection and remember that it's better to apply the sunscreen more often than to use a single application of a sunscreen with a higher SPF number. Always wear sunscreen before applying make up, regardless of your age.

Water. Hydrate your skin with at least 8 glasses per day. Your skin needs moisture and the best way for you to provide that is through water intake and the consumption of water-based foods such as fruits and vegetables.

Food. Limit junk food. Your diet is reflected by your skin, so try to eat a healthy, well balanced diet that includes lots of fresh vegetables and fruit.

The Female Form

The female body is artful with many pleasing curves and angles, denoting a graceful elegance. Good nutrition and exercise are your best strategies for unlocking your *body number*. You may know this already, but it bears repeating. When you select an exercise regimen or program, make sure it's one that's capable of giving you the desired result, and always check with your doctor before beginning any new program.

Take note of how your body responds to certain forms of exercise, and compare that with the ideals we've discussed. When a muscle is worked to the point of fatigue, it responds by getting larger. In this way, the muscle is adapting to handle the increased work load. If the work load increases further, the muscle will enlarge and continue to enlarge as long as the demand exceeds the muscle's ability to provide the required strength.

That means if you are doing an exercise that creates a thigh burn (muscle fatigue), your thigh muscles will respond by getting larger and larger. So if you're concerned about the size of your thighs, knowing this fact may significantly alter which types of exercise you choose to perform.

Always be mindful of the shape you're trying to achieve through exercise. Don't be lured into developing bulky muscles by personal trainers, gym memberships, or home machines that promise they'll shape your body. If you feel a muscle burn and it's a large muscle group like the legs or buttocks, you're likely making those muscles larger. Arms, chest and shoulders tend to be smaller in volume in most women and so these features will not respond and enlarge as quickly as the buttocks and legs. Using smaller weights with higher number reps can tone and firm the arms, shoulders and chest.

Stretching, yoga, Pilates and swimming all produce long, lean muscles that are more consistent with the body style desired by most women. Absolutely everyone benefits from these activities. They emphasize lengthening and toning the muscles while enhancing relaxation along the way.

The elliptical machine, treadmill, or going for a walk or a run are all good sources of increased physical activity. Be aware, though, that running may cause your breasts to prematurely sag if you have fuller breasts. There are suspensory ligaments in your breasts that keep them

The Palmer Code [Francis Palmer MD]

from sagging and the up and down motion of running may weaken them, causing your breasts to sag. If you have larger breasts or have had a breast augmentation surgery, you may not want to run. You can walk or use the elliptical machine or treadmill on a lower setting with minimal incline in order to avoid the jarring up-and-down motion or the muscle burn. Use a lower setting for a longer period of time to achieve the same caloric and aerobic workout without creating bulky muscles.

There's nothing like the feeling of being in the best shape of your life. You look fantastic, you can wear just about anything, and you feel as though you have boundless energy. Experiment with the exercises we just discussed and focus on those you enjoy most. The more you enjoy it, the more likely you are to keep it up. And as we've discussed, the habit is the most important factor. Establishing an excellent regimen that you enjoy puts you one step away from your perfect body.

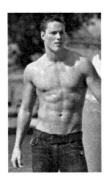

Chapter 10: Men, Unlock Your Palmer Code Body

Unlike the feminine form, the male body is much more utilitarian in design. Built for power and strength, it seems much less complex and more simplistically big, strong and muscular. Because of this emphasis on muscle mass, following good nutrition and exercise will mean quicker results for men. Muscle mass is what essentially regulates metabolism and because men tend to have more muscle mass they also have a higher metabolism. Still, you have to be mindful of what exactly you're striving for, because muscle mass in the wrong places can result in an unbalanced, squat-looking body. Be sure to consult your physician before starting any exercise program.

Unfortunately, unlike women, men have fewer choices when it comes to using clothing to shape the ideal body. There's only so much you can do to add height if you're short and as for the rest—well, it means you'll have to be more keenly focused on nutrition and exercise to bring about your best physical self.

Upper-to-lower body ratio

Consider the two images figures 10-2 and 10-3. The man in figure 10-2 shows the ideal. When measured from the waist, he shows an upper body that is 45% of his

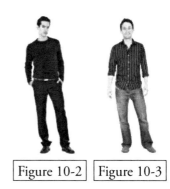

Figure 10-2 | Figure 10-3

overall height, while his lower body makes up the remaining 55%. This means that the legs look longer.

Compare that to the man in figure 10-3, whose upper body looks about 55% of his overall height. Doesn't he look relatively top-heavy as compared to the man in figure 10-2? Doesn't his body look a bit out of balance? A good rule of thumb is to try to avoid letting your upper body look longer than your lower body.

Clothing. Referring again to the two images (figures 10-2 and 10-3) above, the man in Figure 10-3 can readjust his upper-to-lower body ratio by doing nothing more complicated than tucking in his shirt. Often, men leave their shirts out to hide a soft gut. However, the gut remains apparent and the guy just winds up looking sloppy. If you aren't willing to tuck in your shirt, try wearing a tucked-in undershirt with an open button-down shirt that's left out. On the other hand, if your legs are particularly long, the converse is true. With an upper-to-lower body ratio of 45/55, you can leave your shirt un-tucked without looking top-heavy, sloppy or out of balance.

Girth. As a rule, stockier men look shorter, and leaner men look taller. If your upper-to-lower body ratio needs length in the leg, consider slimming down, be it through weight loss or easing away from too much muscle bulk. However, if your legs are particularly long, you can achieve balance by increasing your muscle mass.

Hips and Waist

Hips are not as relevant a feature for men, however they do contribute to an all-important characteristic of the ideal male physique: the V-shape. In men, flat, thin hips make the shoulders, chest and arms appear broader. When coupled with the ideal waist, which is slim and toned without excess fat or skin, the result is the highly sought-after V-shape body style.

Here are some tips to improve these features.

Exercise. Aerobic workouts along with specific exercises designed to tone and firm the waist and hips are the best way to improve this area.

Toning exercises, stretches, or machine exercises specifically designed for this area are all highly recommended.

Nutrition. Eat sensibly to decrease body fat around the midsection.

Clothing. Wear a belt to add visual structure to the hips and emphasize the masculine v-shape.

Legs

Powerful legs add to the ideal male physique, however too much muscle can result in the "squat body" look. Bear in mind that the upper-to-lower body ratio is the most important physical aspect of the body, so while important, heavily-muscled legs are secondary.

Exercise. From weight training to running, the legs respond to a wide range of exercises and physical activities. Anything that causes the thighs to burn will increase the size of your legs. Activities with lighter work loads create toned muscles. Choose your workouts according to your desired leg muscle goal of muscular bulk-up, tone, or de-bulking.

Chest

The third most aesthetically-important body feature for men is the chest. Be mindful of size, shape and tone. V-shaped torsos are perceived as ruggedly masculine.

The chest muscles are made up of the pectoralis major and pectoralis minor muscles. These muscles can be firmed, toned and enlarged depending on how you exercise. You'll want to target these muscles with your workout. Almost universally, men benefit from building up these chest muscles.

Exercise. When you're weight training, focus on the shoulders with bench press and lateral chest curls. Bring the weight into your chest from an outstretched arm position. The chest curl is an excellent way to isolate the chest muscles, while bench presses work the chest, shoulders and arms. Push-ups are another excellent way to build these muscles. For toning and endurance, use speed bag training.

The Palmer Code [Francis Palmer MD]

Clothing. Once again, wearing a belt or tucking in your shirt emphasizes the masculine v-shape, giving the illusion of a broader chest.

Buttocks

The male buttock should be hard, firm and well toned, though somewhat less full and rounded than the female buttocks. For guys, it's a matter of reducing the body fat and increasing the muscular tone of the Gluteus Maximus muscles.

Exercise. Leg curls work the hamstrings and the buttocks, and can be done using free weights or any number of machine exercises that are specifically designed to tighten and firm the buttocks. Isometric exercises that cause the Gluteus Maximus to contract against itself will firm the muscles without causing an increase in size if that is the desired effect. Try standing with your feet apart and forcefully contract the buttocks. Relax and repeat. You can increase the contraction pressure, the hold count and the reps to tailor your workout.

Clothing. Go for the classic: jeans.

Abdomen

This is the one area of the male physique that tells no lies. Six pack abs come from a combination of exercise and ideal body weight, period. Even surgical treatments don't last without proper nutrition and exercise.

Exercise. Yes, you can target your abdominal muscles, but it's pointless if those muscles are hidden under a layer of fat. Go for cardio—running, swimming, cycling—to reduce overall girth. Once your belly begins to disappear, you can focus on targeted work-outs that increase definition. Sit-ups, crunches, leg lifts, or any exercise that focuses on the core will help you achieve a more toned abdomen. Be in tune with what's going on as you work out. You should feel the burn in your abs, not in your back or neck.

[Francis Palmer MD] The Palmer Code

Nutrition. You will find that as your muscle mass increases, you drop the weight faster. Make small changes and make sure they become ingrained habits.

Clothing. The best way to de-emphasize a gut is to wear layered clothing with an open front. For example, wear a t-shirt tucked in with an open button-down over it. Or, wear a dress shirt tucked in with a suit jacket over it—either opened or buttoned. A belt adds structure to the midline.

Shoulders

Men's shoulders give the look of power for the entire upper body. Ideal shoulders are muscular, broad, and thick.

The shoulder muscles can be exercised using strength and muscle-building techniques. The goal is fatigue, which causes hypertrophy of the shoulder muscles. When you work your muscles to the point of complete fatigue (this does not include straining beyond your ability, which can result in muscle tears and injury), the muscles must build up during the rest period that follows your workout. Your body senses that there is an increased demand for additional muscle mass in that area, so it creates additional bulk.

Exercise. Push-ups, pull-ups and chin-ups are excellent exercises for working out the shoulders. When weight training, target the deltoid muscles. Press, bench and curls are good examples of exercises that target these muscles. Do fewer reps with heavier weight to increase muscle mass. Remember that form is everything when using free weights, so get some expert instruction for the most efficient workout possible. Whenever you do bulking exercises, make sure you give yourself the proper repair time so your body has time to build those muscles. A day or two in between work-outs is a good rule of thumb.

Nutrition. If you're looking to increase your muscle mass, your body requires protein to create tissue. This doesn't mean you need to be on an all-protein diet, just make sure you are consuming enough protein for your body to do its job.

The Palmer Code [Francis Palmer MD]

Arms

Like the chest and shoulders, arms reflect power and add to the v-shaped physique. Fortunately, men's arms tend to respond the quickest to focused exercise, building muscle rapidly.

Exercise. Free weights targeting the biceps and forearms are highly effective at enlarging and sculpting the arm muscles. Remember that there are several muscle groups in the arms: biceps and triceps in the upper arm and multiple smaller muscles that make up the forearm. That means you'll have to do several different exercises to work out all of the muscle groups. Use heavier weight with fewer reps to increase the size. Conversely, use lighter weight and more reps if you're more interested in firming and toning the arm muscles. Pushups, pull-ups and chin-ups are good exercises for the arms, as are curls, benches and presses.

Skin

I know, I know. You guys never think about your skin. But take it from me, you should. You don't want to go to all this trouble to create your best body, and then have it all go to waste over negligence. Skin cancer is a very real affliction and it's the fastest-growing cancer in the US. Take time to protect your skin, and you'll stay healthy and look great.

Sun. Avoid excess sun exposure, including sun tan booths.

Water. Hydrate yourself by drinking a minimum of eight glasses of water per day.

Nutrition. Avoid junk food. That's just another way to introduce free radicals and all kinds of damaging influences. Go for fruits and vegetables instead, which carry vitamins and moisture to the skin.

Care. Use high quality skin care products that help provide protection and much-needed moisture. Use an SPF 30 or higher UVA and UVB sunscreen if you're going outside.

[Francis Palmer MD] The Palmer Code

The Male Physique

When you're at your physical best, you feel like a powerhouse and you look terrific. It's worthwhile to put the extra effort into bringing your body to its best physical condition. Start with incremental changes, increasing the frequency of your workouts and tightening your nutritional regimen. Work toward being the one in the room with the coveted v-shape. Guaranteed, whatever might be keeping you from that now—whatever procrastination is getting in the way—can't top the feeling of being at your physical best.

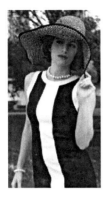

Chapter 11: Supporting Factors

The supporting factors play a role in *your number* within the *Palmer Code*, which are defined within the formula for the *outer you*:

Physical Features (80%) + Grooming (10%) + Style (10%) = Outer You (100%)

Breaking it down even further, let's look at what comprises the physical features:

Face (50%) + Body (30%) + Skin (10%) + Hair (10%) = Physical Features (100%)

Together, skin and hair contribute 20% to *your number* for physical features, so it's important to take good care of them.

Skin

The skin is the largest organ of the body and perhaps the most often overlooked. It contributes in multiple ways to *your number* and is represented within your *face number*, your *body number* and as a separate supporting element of your *physical appearance*, so it's well worth your attention.

The Palmer Code   [Francis Palmer MD]

Smooth, firm, youthful-looking skin is attractive, and it's something you should strive to achieve. Really, it's just a matter of prevention. The goal is to protect your skin from age and damage, because we start out lives with fresh, beautiful baby skin. Some of us then proceed to allow our environment to change the texture, quality and appearance. Let's put a stop to that right now.

Here are the various components of the skin (table 11-1) and their relative importance (100 points possible):

SKIN	
Degree of firmness and tone (loose skin vs. taut)	30 points
Texture	20 points
Consistent pigment	18 points
Amount of wrinkles and folds	17 points
Degree of fatty tissue	10 points
Prevalence of blemishes and contour defects (scars, acne, etc.)	5 points
Total	**100 points**

Table 11-1

For this evaluation, remove all makeup and analyze your skin in accordance with the factors in Table 11-1 above. Remember that this evaluation is more about what you don't have—interfering factors such as blemishes—than anything else. The closer you are to that baby soft skin you were born with, the better. Record your points.

Unlike a perfect nose, full set of lips or the ideal cheeks, we are pretty much

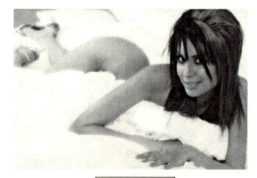

Figure 11-2

all born with beautiful skin. It's the one feature that we are all given close to ideal, so what happens to change things?

As mentioned throughout this book, we ignore the skin, plain and simple. In our teens, we over-expose the skin to the sun or use tanning booths, we don't eat properly, or we ignore quality skin care products. As a result, somewhere in our thirties, the skin starts to age prematurely, showing signs of wrinkling, roughened texture, dull color and loss of elasticity and tone. These changes simply accelerate as we get older, until we look at our skin and attempt to halt or reverse the damage. I think that's the wrong approach whether it's the skin of the face or the body. We should start thinking about protecting our skin as teens.

I have mentioned these simple rules for beautiful skin throughout the book, but they warrant repeating.

1. Avoid excess UV exposure from the sun or tanning booths.
2. Use a quality sunscreen with UVA and UVB protection every day.
3. Maintain a healthy diet, limiting junk food (this also helps control acne).
4. Hydrate with a minimum of 8 glasses of water per day.
5. Establish good skin hygiene and cleansing regimens, avoiding harsh abrasives and chemical exfoliants.

If these habits are established as a routine for our teens to follow throughout their lives, the vast majority of them will maintain their beautiful skin well into their 60's and beyond. If you're already beyond your teens, just know that it's never too late to establish excellent habits.

Hair

Hair is the final component of your physical features. Like the skin, hair contributes to *your number* in multiple ways not only as part of your physical features but also as a component of your *face number*. In this case we're not just talking about your hairstyle. We're also looking at the actual fullness of hair that you have, the hairline, the size of the exposed forehead and the degree of thinning hair (table 11-2).

The Palmer Code [Francis Palmer MD]

HAIR	
Fullness of hair	50 points
Hair/forehead ratio (degree of thinning)	50 points

Table 11-2

If you have full, thick hair with a forehead that is a third the distance from the front hairline to the bottom of your chin, then give yourself the full 100 points possible.

Chances are you know whether you have a receding hairline, your forehead is over-exposed, or if your hair is thinning. If these are present, deduct points from your hair score.

Note that nowadays baldness has come into style. So if you're thinning up top, this is your day. In fact, ruggedly-handsome features are emphasized by a shaved head. Just be aware that the style to follow is the shaved-down or quarter-inch trim, not the legendary "comb-over" that men have been attempting for centuries. The former is a show of male confidence; the latter isn't.

That said, there are still a number of ways that men and women can deal with baldness, from hair weaves to topical creams and pills, to wigs and toupees. If you feel strongly that you want to pursue a full head of hair, talk to your doctor about the strategy that's right for you.

Other Outer You Components

Grooming (table 11-3) includes hairstyle and make-up and plays a significant role in the *Palmer Code*. Here again, it's one of those components that is only relevant when it's distracting. For example, suppose you came across a very handsome man, but he's been on a camping trip and it's apparent that he hasn't taken a shower in a week. His *number* would decrease accordingly. But grooming can have a more subtle effect as well. The right hairstyle can accentuate your best features, while the wrong one can compete with them.

[Francis Palmer MD] The Palmer Code

POINT SYSTEM FOR GROOMING

WOMEN		MEN	
Hairstyle	50 points	Hairstyle	50 points
Make up	30 points	Clean and neat	50 points
Clean and neat	20 points		
Total	**100 points**	**Total**	**100 points**

Table 11-3

A good method to determine your score is to take a digital photo of your face and calculate your *face number*. When objectively analyzing your face, does your hairstyle accentuate or detract from the "big three" facial features? If it does, determine by how much? Deduct points accordingly.

We discussed how different hairstyles affect your features in previous chapters. I recommend you take the time to really explore how you can choose a style that frames the top aesthetic facial features.

If you have ideal or close to ideal facial features, you can wear almost any hairstyle. Off the face, pulled, back, cropped short—it doesn't matter much. If, on the other hand, your facial features are less than ideal (especially the cheeks), think about hairstyles that frame the forehead and face. The picture in figure 11-3 is a good example of hair that frames the face well and softens the cheeks.

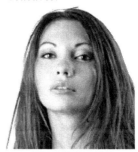

Figure 11-3

Makeup can either accentuate or detract from your facial features. As with the hair, try taking a digital picture of your face after you've finished your makeup and calculate your *face number*. Does your makeup technique accentuate or detract from the "big three" facial features? If it highlights your features, give yourself the full points possible. If not, deduct accordingly.

Grooming is certainly all about being clean and neat. If you're well put-together, go ahead and take the total points possible.

Style

This category includes clothing, color palette and accessories (table 11-4).

STYLE	
Style and clothing	50 points
Color palette	25 points
Accessories	25 points

Table 11-4

It's no surprise that certain clothes make you feel more beautiful than others. You've heard the term "the clothes make the man". As previously stated, the right color and style of clothing will improve *your number* just as surely as the wrong clothes will decrease it. When conducting the self-evaluation, give yourself points if your clothing, color palette and accessories reflect current trends. If you dress in sweats every day, or if you are wearing the same shirt you were wearing fifteen years ago, deduct points.

You probably already know whether you have a keen sense of style. For most people, it's a matter of putting in the effort. The more you look at fashion magazines, taking note of people you believe are well-dressed, the keener your sense of style becomes. If you feel you're lacking, a good rule of thumb is that it's often best to default to a more conservative look and approach.

The Outer you

You now have all the information you need to calculate the *outer you*. This comprises 60% of *your number* within the *Palmer Code number*. In the next phase, we'll delve deeper inside—literally—and take a look at the *inner you* which contributes the remaining 40% to *your number*.

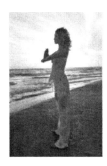

Chapter 12: The Inner You

The Mysteries of Attraction

Beauty and attraction have always gone hand in hand. In fact, the human response to beauty can be downright primal. This is true sexuality to be certain, but attraction isn't always about sex. Simply stated, attraction is anything that attracts. You may be attracted to a beautiful painting, a river, a mentor whose accomplishments you admire, a piano concerto, a basketful of puppies... anything. This is what I call the inner light, that thing inside of you that is the *inner you*.

If you don't believe the *inner you* has much to do with your beauty, consider this: there are supermodels and there are superstars. A supermodel might look good on the runway or in pictures, but it takes a certain degree of personality to become a superstar. Some supermodels such as Heidi Klum can make that transition and as a result she has become both. Consider this point; for the most part, when we see celebrities onscreen, in interviews or situations where we can observe and respond to their essence, that's when we get hooked and keep coming back for more. There's nothing headier than being in the presence of someone who is both beautiful on the outside and fascinating on the inside. This is the core of attraction.

• • •

"Simply stated, attraction is anything that attracts."

• • •

The Palmer Code [Francis Palmer MD]

Before we get into the code of attraction and the *inner you*, I'd like to pause and ask you to take a mental snapshot of this very moment. Observe what's going on inside you even as you read this. Now ask yourselves the following questions as they pertain to you *right now*:

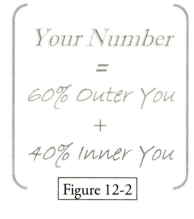

Figure 12-2

1. How is your health?
2. How much sleep did you get last night?
3. When was the last time you had sex?
4. What does your home environment look like (pleasing to look at or an eyesore filled with visual reminders of chores)?
5. What was the last thing you ate?
6. When was the last time you moved your body to the point of sweat?
7. When was the last time you engaged in spiritual activity?
8. What is your current social standing?
9. Is there anything in your life that you think you need but are not getting?
10. When was the last time you did something creative?
11. How are your relationships with friends and family?

I hope you answered most, if not all, of these questions in the positive but regardless, what we're about to discuss is not so much about how you responded; the point is actually in the asking. You see, there's a lot of power in posing questions to yourself. By creating a habit of turning your awareness inward you become more tuned in to the *inner you* and you can strengthen that light just as surely as you build muscles when you exercise regularly. We're going to get into the mechanics of that in the next chapter, "Unlocking the Inner You." For now I just want you to keep the questions in the back of your mind as we go through the next several pages, and we'll come back to them again at the end of this section.

Components of the Inner You

The Inner You = Emotional Well-Being + Physical Well-Being

Remember the garden we created in Chapter 1? Suppose for a moment that you wanted to invite the neighbors over one evening to celebrate the renovation. You hang Chinese lanterns and put on some soothing, lovely music. The flowers are soft and fragrant, the creek is clear and cool and winking with fireflies.

The first family arrives, but they hardly notice the garden setting because they are bickering with one another. You show them around

"When you feel a sense of bliss and find joy in the things around you, the inner you shines and you are more attractive."

and they pause their sparring long enough to complain that the creek and the birds are awfully noisy—and speaking of noise, do you realize what they had to put up with while you were creating this garden? All those trucks delivering materials and that sawing and hammering when the gazebo went up!

Then the second family arrives. They are at least in good temper, however they admit that they've been passing around a cold and are congested, red-eyed and slow-moving. You're thinking, *that poor family, but didn't they have a cold the last time I saw them? No, wait; that was the stomach flu.* You seat them in the gazebo where they won't have to move around much and you make a beeline to the sink to wash your hands.

The Palmer Code [Francis Palmer MD]

Finally, the third family arrives. They look around in amazement at the fairytale setting that, having had to deal with the bickerers and the sickies, you've all but forgotten about. Watching the third family take to the garden with joy refreshes your own sense of delight: The children chase fireflies and cool their toes in the creek. The wife is taking in the luscious scent of the jasmine as the husband asks you for pointers on how he might bring a little magic into his own garden.

• • •

"Take note of who you are bringing into your garden."

• • •

Based solely on this experience, which family do you want to invite back?

Once again, the garden illustrates aspects of the *Palmer Code*. This time, the human aspect represents components of the *inner you*. When you are sick or when you are emotionally unsettled, *your number* sinks. The converse is also true. When you feel a sense of bliss and can take joy in the things around you, the *inner you* shines, and you are more attractive.

These families are just people you invited over, aren't they? They don't necessarily reflect you, right? Well, yes and no. Suppose you spent a year on a deserted island with the bickering, complaining family or with the hypochondriacs. Now, contrast that with the thought of spending a year isolated with the family that exhibits a natural joie de vivre. Don't you think that by the end of that year, you might have taken on at least some of the qualities of those people with whom you spent all that time? Consider that for a moment, and then ask yourself, right now, who you've invited into the garden that is your life.

Emotional Well-Being and the Palmer Code

In a way, emotional well-being is a balance of spirit. It's a reflection of your emotions, your mental health and the way you perceive yourself not only as an individual but in the broader context of society. The way you interact with strangers, friends and family members reflect the state of your relationships. Your relationship with God, or the spiritual acuity that forms the basis of your beliefs, also contributes to your emotional well-being.

Stress, as I'm sure you know, is a significant factor in you emotional well-being. Even more important is how you handle the stress. For example, suppose two women are stuck in a traffic jam. The first woman is tapping her fingers, sipping her hot coffee even though she's already getting the sense that she ought to get to a restroom soon and she's wishing ardently that everyone would just *move*. She grows more frustrated when she sees that the cars in front of her are taking delayed, slinky-like intervals as they move forward. She lays on the horn and in her agitation she spills coffee on her blouse, burning her and setting her up to look all the more ridiculous for that meeting she should be walking into right now if she wasn't stuck in this horrible, horrible traffic!

The second woman sees the traffic, sees that some cars are moving forward sluggishly and decides that the situation is what it is and there's not much she can do about it. She phones her office (using the hands-free, voice-activated utility, of course) to let them know she'll be late, setting clear expectations of her situation among her colleagues. Then she switches on an audio book that she's been enjoying and practices her facial exercises to enhance her excellent cheeks. As she sits in that very same traffic jam, it occurs to her that this is actually a pleasant stolen moment.

Of the two women above, which do you suppose scores higher in emotional well-being, resulting in a higher *inner you* number?

Environment can also contribute to your emotional state. You probably spend a significant amount of time in your home and place of work. How do you fell when you look around?

| The Palmer Code | [Francis Palmer MD]

Physical Well-Being and the Palmer Code

There are many facets to being physically healthy. There's illness and chronic afflictions on one end of the spectrum and athletic physical conditioning and healthy eating habits on the other end. Many people try to force optimum physical rhythms by loading up on caffeine in the morning and alcohol at night. I'm not saying you should never drink coffee or wine—not by any means—but you should be in tune with what's going on inside your body.

Consider the following scenario: Two 43 year-old men each have *Palmer Code numbers* of 88. One man is in good overall health, exercises regularly and eats sensibly. The other doesn't exercise and is exhibiting early signs of hypertension and high cholesterol. How long before the second man sees a decrease in his **inner you** with corresponding **decreases in his outer you and whole you numbers?**

As the hypertension takes its toll on his energy level and darkens his mood, he begins to have the occasional headache. He's weak, so he doesn't feel like exercising which only slows him down and causes him to feel out of shape. His mood and fitness level spiral downward. The end result is that he's feeling less confident and soon after, he is less outgoing. With each increment of this spiral, his *number* ticks down, down, by small but inevitable amounts. We all know that when we have a cold or the flu, we feel lousy and look pretty awful as well.

Emotional Well-Being (50%) + Physical Well-Being (50%) = Inner You (100%)

Shining Your Light

Remember that your personality, your inner essence, is affected by many different factors such as personal relationships at home, work and with God. Your emotional and physical health influence how you

[Francis Palmer MD] The Palmer Code

feel about yourself. You as an individual are unique. There is no other person exactly like you. What makes you who and what you are can't be defined solely by your external appearance. Your feelings, emotions and experiences all contribute to make the *total you* and *your number.*

When you can turn your attention inward and take a clear, objective reading of what's going on inside, you can help the *inner you* blossom. In the next chapter we'll discuss how to do exactly that.

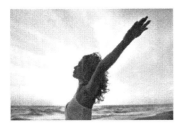

Chapter 13: Unlocking the Inner You

We've discussed how your emotional and physical well-being can affect how attractive you are from the inside out. Let's look at ways that you can use this information to take control of the impression you leave on others and more importantly, how you feel inside your own skin.

I'm going to pose some questions again, but this time, I'd like you to get out a pencil and track you points for each answer. When you answer the questions on the following pages, you achieve three distinct goals:

- Thoughtful analysis of these aspects of your life
- Highlight areas of strength as well as those that require your attention
- Present a recipe for meaningful change

When you answer the following yes-or-no questions, assign yourself points according to the following scale (table 13-1):

Your answer	Points
Absolutely	5
Yes	4
Sort of	3
Not sure	2
Not really	1
No	0

| The Palmer Code | [Francis Palmer MD]

Physical Well-Being Analysis

Are you in overall good health and free of acute illness?
> Absolutely! (5 pts) Yes (4 pts) Sort of (3 pts) Not sure (2 pts)
> Not really (1 pt) No (0 pts)

Are you free of heart disease, hypertension (high blood pressure), diabetes, hepatitis or HIV?
> Absolutely! (5 pts) Yes (4 pts) Sort of (3 pts) Not sure (2 pts)
> Not really (1 pt) No (0 pts)

Are you free of cancer, rheumatoid arthritis, or any chronic or systemic illness?
> Absolutely! (5 pts) Yes (4 pts) Sort of (3 pts) Not sure (2 pts)
> Not really (1 pt) No (0 pts)

Do you strive to eat healthy foods?
> Absolutely! (5 pts) Yes (4 pts) Sort of (3 pts) Not sure (2 pts)
> Not really (1 pt) No (0 pts)

Is your weight less than your ideal weight plus 15%? (see reference chart Appendix B)
> Absolutely! (5 pts) Yes (4 pts) Sort of (3 pts) Not sure (2 pts)
> Not really (1 pt) No (0 pts)

Do you engage in exercise or some other strenuous activity lasting at least 30 minutes three times a week or more?
> Absolutely! (5 pts) Yes (4 pts) Sort of (3 pts) Not sure (2 pts)
> Not really (1 pt) No (0 pts)

Are you free of significant known health risk factors, including high cholesterol (total over 200), high blood glucose, or borderline high blood pressure (140/90)?
> Absolutely! (5 pts) Yes (4 pts) Sort of (3 pts) Not sure (2 pts)
> Not really (1 pt) No (0 pts)

[Francis Palmer MD] **The Palmer Code**

Do you have a basic understanding of how different types of foods such as fruits and vegetables impact your health?
> Absolutely! (5 pts) Yes (4 pts) Sort of (3 pts) Not sure (2 pts) Not really (1 pt) No (0 pts)

Do you have basic knowledge of the benefits of vitamins, minerals, and supplements?
> Absolutely! (5 pts) Yes (4 pts) Sort of (3 pts) Not sure (2 pts) Not really (1 pt) No (0 pts)

Do you have a basic understanding of how body metabolism is affected by food type, number of meals per day, total calories consumed, and total calories burned?
> Absolutely! (5 pts) Yes (4 pts) Sort of (3 pts) Not sure (2 pts) Not really (1 pt) No (0 pts)

Tally your points for the physical well-being analysis, and enter your score here:_____

Emotional Well-Being Analysis

Would you describe yourself as basically a happy person?
> Absolutely! (5 pts) Yes (4 pts) Sort of (3 pts) Not sure (2 pts) Not really (1 pt) No (0 pts)

Do you feel that you have a nice life?
> Absolutely! (5 pts) Yes (4 pts) Sort of (3 pts) Not sure (2 pts) Not really (1 pt) No (0 pts)

Do you look forward to seeing and interacting with your family?
> Absolutely! (5 pts) Yes (4 pts) Sort of (3 pts) Not sure (2 pts) Not really (1 pt) No (0 pts)

| The Palmer Code | [Francis Palmer MD]

Can you think of at least one person that you consider a close friend with whom you can share portions of your life?
> Absolutely! (5 pts) Yes (4 pts) Sort of (3 pts) Not sure (2 pts) Not really (1 pt) No (0 pts)

Do you feel fulfilled and appreciated at work?
> Absolutely! (5 pts) Yes (4 pts) Sort of (3 pts) Not sure (2 pts) Not really (1 pt) No (0 pts)

When you're in a serious relationship, are you committed to your partner and the relationship?
> Absolutely! (5 pts) Yes (4 pts) Sort of (3 pts) Not sure (2 pts) Not really (1 pt) No (0 pts)

Do you believe in God or a higher spiritual authority/existence?
> Absolutely! (5 pts) Yes (4 pts) Sort of (3 pts) Not sure (2 pts) Not really (1 pt) No (0 pts)

Do you have a positive opinion of yourself?
> Absolutely! (5 pts) Yes (4 pts) Sort of (3 pts) Not sure (2 pts) Not really (1 pt) No (0 pts)

Most of the time, do you feel calm at work and at home?
> Absolutely! (5 pts) Yes (4 pts) Sort of (3 pts) Not sure (2 pts) Not really (1 pt) No (0 pts)

Are you generally excited to try new things and seek new experiences?
> Absolutely! (5 pts) Yes (4 pts) Sort of (3 pts) Not sure (2 pts) Not really (1 pt) No (0 pts)

Tally your points for the emotional well-being analysis, and enter your score here:_____

Understanding Your Inner You Number

At first glance, the *inner you* may seem like an abstract idea of how you feel. However, within physical and emotional well-being are aspects of

[Francis Palmer MD] **The Palmer Code**

our daily lives that have long been recognized as important contributors to perceived quality of life. We will now take a closer look at some aspects of the *inner you* and just as we did with the *outer you*, we will use the *Palmer Code* to prioritize the various *inner you* components.

In the **Physical Well Being** self-examination, the questions were grouped into the following general categories (table 13-2):

Categories	Questions
Physical Health and Possible Risk Factors	1-4
Body Habitus	5
Activity Level	6
Nutrition & Eating Habits	7-10

Table 13-2

As you go back and look at your score within each of the categories mentioned above, take note of answers rating a score of 3 or lower, which indicate areas that require further self-examination. By doing this, you'll get an idea what may require your attention, further education, or improvement. Say, for instance that you have three low scores within the nutrition and eating habits category. This may suggest that you should learn some basic information about nutrition and the influence that food and metabolism have on your overall health and your body.

The **Emotional Well-Being** categories are as follows (table 13-3):

Categories	Questions
Emotion & Attitude	11-12
Relationships	13-17
Self-Perception	18
Stress & Coping	19-20

Table 13-3

Just as you did with your Physical Well-Being scores, those within the Emotional Well-Being section can guide your self-analysis and improvement. Once again examine your answers within each category

135

and if you've answered a question with a score of 3 or less, take a closer look at that aspect of your life. Only through focused self-examination can you identify areas of concern that may require your attention or improvement.

Now that you have identified your areas of strengths and weaknesses, how can you prioritize these categories to effect meaningful change? Turns out, there is a specific way to look at this. A simple way to nurture the *inner you* is to examine whether your needs are being met. A good representation of this is Maslow's Hierarchy of Needs, proposed by psychologist Abraham Maslow in 1943 (figure 13-2).

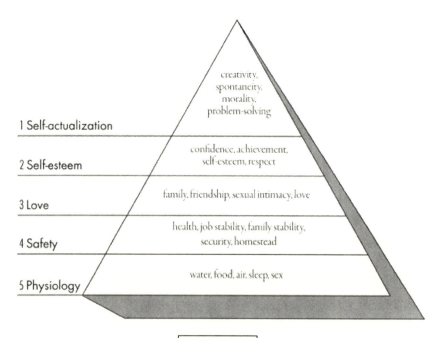

Figure 13-2

This pyramid is a portrayal of Maslow's Hierarchy of Needs. Maslow believed that humans must satisfy basic needs first—portrayed at the base of the pyramid—before we can truly raise ourselves to new levels and meet more evolved needs. However, once we've moved up

[Francis Palmer MD] **The Palmer Code**

the pyramid, we easily return to the highest level we've achieved. That means if you have reached self-actualization but you suffer a health setback, you will tend to the health issue but continue operating at the self-actualization level. The higher you step through the pyramid, the brighter the *inner you* and the greater your beauty shines.

Looking at these basic needs, once you have food, water and shelter, personal safety is the next priority. This includes physical health, emotional health and stable enriching relationships, whether they be at work, home, or of a higher spiritual nature. To assess your level of personal safety, go back and look at your scores for questions 1-10 and 13-17. If your score for the first 10 questions indicate that you may need improvement, this may entail medical intervention, adopting a healthy eating philosophy, embracing a consistent exercise regimen, or the incorporation of nutritional supplements. If your scores for questions 13-17 indicate that your relationships need further work, this may require professional help to assess your personal relationships and provide further instruction on ways that you can change them in a positive and fulfilling manner.

Next on the priority list is self-esteem, which is addressed in questions 11, 12 and 18. It's sometimes tough to have a healthy perception of ourselves in today's hectic, fast-paced society, but it's nevertheless extremely important for you to maintain a strong sense of your self-worth and value. If your answers suggest this is an area in which you can improve, there are many steps that you can take.

First, consider this simple exercise. Tell yourself five times a day, *"I'm happy, I love myself and I deserve goods things in my life."* Don't just mouth the words, but say it like you mean it.

Find simple things in which you can excel. Help others at work or in your community because a great way for you to feel good about yourself is in the service of others. There are many organizations that would love to have you volunteer your time and efforts assisting those who are in need.

Finally, at the top of the needs priority is self-actualization—through creativity and spontaneity. When you feel secure and nurtured, your creative juices begin to flow. Think for a moment. What could be a better project with which to hone your creativity than…you? Your self-development and improvement.

If you've been paying attention, you may have noticed that I haven't mentioned questions 19 and 20 which deal with stress and your coping mechanisms. It' been said that *the only constant is change.* Simply put, this means that every aspect of our lives is in a constant state of flux, as nothing stays the same forever. Our age, our appearance, relationships, society, technology…everything changes and will continue to do so until the end of time. Does that seem unsettling or scary? How we deal with stress and how we cope with the inevitable changes in our lives has a huge impact on how we feel and look. For that reason, I have left stress and how to cope with it as the final *inner you* component.

Stress

I know what you're thinking. What does stress have to do with beauty? The answer: plenty.

One of the biggest *inner you* zappers is stress. Stress can take its toll physically as well as emotionally: it can cause your hair to fall out, skin to dry, blood pressure to rise and can turn you into an emotional train wreck. Physical conditions such as coronary artery disease, peptic ulcer, and mental illness are often stress-related.

When you think about it, stress is usually tied to fear. You may be experiencing a fear of failure, such as a worry that you might be late, miss a deadline, or let someone down. Fears that lead to stress may also culminate as fear of the unknown, fear of rejection, fear of conflict, fear of risk or trust, insecurity, or inability to cope with new or changing circumstances.

As humans, we are constantly being put to the test by our relationships, environment, and circumstances. A natural tendency is to eliminate stress by creating an optimum environment. You only get close to people you can trust, or you repeatedly go to the same places where the food is reliable, the setting is predictable and the circumstances are always the same. But is it realistic to believe you can always control your circumstances? Isn't life bound to throw you a curve ball sooner or later? Your best weapon is not to cocoon yourself inside a predictable, reliable world. People who are free from stress are those who know how to cope with change.

To better cope with stress, it's important to take a careful look at how it manifests—and it's not always bad. A good example of this is physical stress. When you're exercising, that slight push you give yourself is what gives your body the most benefits. The same is true of emotional stress.

Consider the three levels of stress:

- **Eustress**—This is the *optimum,* stress-free level. In the eustress zone, you are actively thinking, creating, stretching, exerting, or learning. Be it mentally or physically or both, you are progressing.
- **Distress**—This is the lowest level where we begin to feel stressed. It can show itself in the form of frustration, dissatisfaction, boredom or even fatigue.
- **High stress**—High stress is the least favorable *inner you* zone. In this zone, you have abandoned your inner bliss and are reacting to circumstances using irrational problem-solving actions.

In just about any capacity, going to the eustress level will counteract the effects of high stress or distress. Think about it: Is there any situation where stressing out is helpful? Even if you're being chased by a bear, your best bet is to employ calm, clear thinking while you act.

The eustress zone means you are calm, yet active and effective. You take action when your actions make a difference and you peacefully accept the situation when they do not. In eustress, you're active; but when in distress or high stress, you are *re*-active.

The Palmer Code [Francis Palmer MD]

Here are some examples of common situations and typical active and reactive responses (table 13-4):

SITUATION	ACTIVE	REACTIVE
Missing a deadline on the job	Accept the situation, inform relevant team members, and work at a reasonable pace	Worry about the situation and alternate between paralysis and heroic spurts of productivity; avoid team members
Children screaming and crying	Remain calm; take action if possible, accept if not	Scream back
Relaxing	Yoga	Watching television
Rejection	Accept and move on	Make arguments inside your head, worry, assume lowered sense of self worth

In an active, eustress mode, you are calm and in control. In distress or high stress modes, the illusion is that you are in control, but you're really not. You're in a passive, *reactive* state of mind. To keep stress at bay, you must be in the habit of keeping an active, peaceful mind.

So how do you achieve this? Exercise, meditation, yoga and simply being aware are all useful coping mechanisms. When you feel yourself enter an alarm state because a stressor has triggered a stress reaction, turn your awareness inward and watch closely. Often if you can focus on your own reaction and not the stressor itself, you can maintain an active, peaceful state of mind and deal with the situation with more control.

The way you handle stress is such a simple, easily-controlled behavior and yet that single habit has a tremendous impact on your emotional well-being, your physical body and ultimately, *your number*.

[Francis Palmer MD] The Palmer Code

The next two pages have diagrams (figures 13-3 and 13-4) depicting not only the typical stress response, they also show you how you can teach yourself to control the effect stress has on your body. Remember, learning to effectively cope with stress is an exercise and as with any exercise, the more you practice it the more proficient you become.

Your personal stress response (figure 13-3) defines the way you handle stress. In that moment when you encounter a stressor, your personal stress response puts you in an active or reactive mode. If you're reactive, you won't even think about it; you'll just react. If you're active, you'll have a sense of heightened awareness but your sense of well-being is not affected, no matter how dire the circumstances.

A passive/reactive personal stress response gets filtered through your brain, engaging the hypothalamus and pituitary gland, sending signals to your adrenal glands and your entire sympathetic nervous system. Together, they create a physical response in your body. This can mean sweats, an elevated heart rate, high blood pressure, respiration, dilated pupils and a host of "juices" your body secretes in order to cope—juices that can take their toll on you over time.

Conversely, your personal relaxation message (figure 13-4) results in the opposite effect. You induce your own relaxation message and you interpret that through your relaxation response. This sends "quiet down" signals to the pituitary gland, the hypothalamus, the adrenal gland and the sympathetic nervous system.

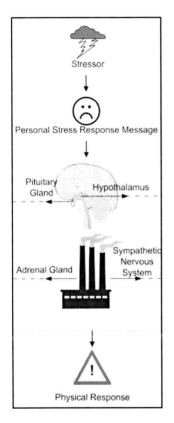

Stress Response in the Human Body

Figure 13-3

141

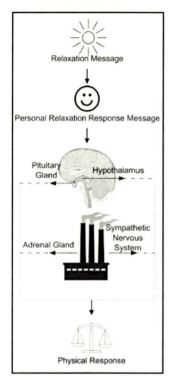

Relaxation in the Human Body

Figure 13-4

The result? Easy breathing, lower heart rate, decreased blood pressure decrease and eased muscle tension. Your personality controls how you interpret sources of stress and how often you seek relaxation. These habits have a profound effect on both your mental and your physical well-being.

Learn ways to develop the habit of creating relaxation messages that you can do throughout the day. The more often you practice, the easier it gets. Soon you'll find that relaxation—not stress—is your default state of being.

Habits

The most direct path to bringing the *inner you* to its full potential is to establish good *inner you* habits. Healthy eating, appropriate exercise and relaxation should be part of your daily routine. My up-and-coming books, *The Palmer Code Diet* and *The Palmer Code Exercise Guide*, will provide you with more specific guidelines if you are interested in improving those aspects of your life.

For now, the most important thing you can do is perfect your habits. Habits are everything. Relaxation habits, healthy eating and consistent exercise are all achievable when you focus on integrating them into your daily routine. Even modest changes can have profound effects over the long term. By automatically reaching for healthy foods first and by being in the habit of regularly moving your body, you experience the first major successes. The rest is fine-tuning.

Now that you have learned how to maximize the *inner you*, the next few chapters will examine how the *Palmer Code* can be used to maintain *your number* and influence your relationships.

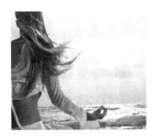

Chapter 14: Achieve and Maintain Your Number and Best Self

Congratulations! You've learned all the components of the *Palmer Code* and have calculated *your number.*

In order to achieve your best self, you're probably going to have to develop some new habits. This might be as simple as putting on sunscreen every morning, or it might be a sweeping overhaul of your approach to nutrition and exercise. First let's take a look at some of the habits that will bring about the ideal you and then we'll talk about how to make them a seamless part of your routine.

Maintaining Your Number for the Face

1. **Avoid sun exposure.** The quickest way to age your face is to bake under the sun or in a tanning booth, and that means lines, wrinkles, and rough, sagging skin. Ladies, get in the habit of applying sunscreen under your make up in the morning. Even if you don't plan on spending a lot of time outside, should the situation arise, you'll be covered. Apply UVA and UVB sunscreen to your face and chest every single day.
2. **Facial exercises.** Do these every single day. You can do them in the shower, in your car during your commute, or any time you have a quiet moment. You will maintain muscle tone and will have a firm, more youthful-looking face.

The Palmer Code [Francis Palmer MD]

3. **Eat right.** Avoid junk food, which is a playground for free radicals and counter-nutrients. Avoid sugar, salt, and saturated fats. Opt instead for healthy fruits and vegetables, which are rich in both nutrients and water. It's the best, most effective way of injecting all-natural vitamins into your system.

4. **Water.** Moisturize from the inside before you moisturize on the outside. Drink at least eight glasses a day, and keep after those fruits and vegetables.

5. **Care.** Use high quality skin care products and treatments to maintain fresh, youthful skin. It's much easier to maintain beautiful skin than to try to re-create it later, once the damage has already occurred. Ideally, start in your late teens or twenties and continue throughout your life.

6. **Style.** Take time to apply make up in such a way that best accentuates the features you want to emphasize, those that carry the most relevance in the *Palmer Code.*

7. **Hygiene.** Take time to groom your face, hair, and teeth.

Maintaining Your Number for the Body

1. **Exercise.** I'll say it again: Exercise! Establish this habit now and continue it for life. Be mindful of the types of exercises that will accentuate your body to its fullest potential. For women, stretching exercises such as yoga and Pilates should be a staple. Men should focus on more muscle-building routines targeting the shoulder, arms and chest to create the classic v-shaped body.

2. **Clothing.** Take extra time to wear clothes that flatter your body. Remember dark clothes and straight lines are more slimming. The most important visual factor is the upper-to-lower body ratio, so dress accordingly.

Maintaining Your Skin
(Same Principles As The Face)

1. **Sunscreen.** Wear it every time you might be going outside. If you're at the beach or you expect prolonged exposure for any other reason, apply it often. Also, opt for self-tanners over sunbathing or tanning beds.
2. **Hydrate.** Drink eight or more glasses of water a day, and eat lots of fruits and vegetables.

Maintaining Your Hair

1. **Groom.** Brush your hair daily. Wash and moisturize your hair often.
2. **Supplements.** Nutritional supplements such as niacin can enhance hair growth. Take them regularly to get the full benefit and consider medical treatments to regain hair growth such as Rogaine®, Propecia® and hair transplantation if further effects are desired.
3. **Style.** Wear a hairstyle that frames your eyes and flatters your face.

Maintaining Your Emotional Health
and Your Number within the Inner You

1. **Joy.** Practice being happy. Tell yourself every day that you are fortunate to be alive and find something to be happy about during that day.
2. **Reduce stress.** Meditate, relax and embrace change. Life is all about change, so you might as well embrace it as a way of keeping things new, fresh and exciting.
3. **Love.** Maintain healthy relationships on all levels: spiritual, personal and professional. It's easier to cope with life when you have support.

The Palmer Code [Francis Palmer MD]

4. **Kindness.** Try to be a good person and you'll feel better about yourself, your life and how you fit into society. Remember to be kind to everyone including yourself. Learn to love and forgive yourself just as you would others.

5. **Indulge.** Do something fresh that brings you extreme satisfaction: go back to school, or take a trip somewhere you've always wanted to go. Allow yourself to live and thoroughly enjoy life. It's why we are here.

6. **Ask for help.** If you are depressed, have self-esteem issues, problems with relationships, or feel powerless over any aspect of your life, consider talking to a professional who can help get you through it. There's no reason or benefit in trying to tough it out on your own.

Maintaining Your Physical Health and Your Number within the Inner You

1. **Exercise.** Notice how frequently this topic comes up in the *Palmer Code*? That's for a reason. Exercise is good therapy for just about every aspect of your life. Adopt a reasonable exercise program that you can live with and actually maintain over the years. Think of physical activity—tennis, running, skiing—as an enjoyable social event. It's a good attitude that will help you remain active for many years.

2. **Eat sensibly.** Diet is a four-letter word that rarely works. Why? Because it's natural to hate something when you're feeling deprived and the mere fact that you're dieting means you're depriving yourself of something. Learn to appreciate good, healthy foods and the weight will regulate itself.

3. **Supplements.** Take vitamins and minerals to make sure you're getting the proper nutrition.

4. **Water.** Your body needs water to keep the engines cool, so drink it throughout the day. Drink even more water when you're exercising.

5. **See your physician.** Get routine physical checkups and screening examinations. It's much easier to nip a problem in the bud if it's caught in the early stages. Your doctor will check for hypertension, high cholesterol, heart disease and other afflictions that are all too common. Screening tests save lives, so be sure to get them on a regular basis.

Establishing the Habit

It may seem that this chapter lists many things you'll want to incorporate into your life and that's good. Think of it as a mirror that reflects your ideal self. It's your job to create that self. The key is to develop habits that maintain *your number*.

If you've ever developed a good habit, you know how satisfying it is. Perhaps you've taken up running. One day you're saying, "Yeah, I keep meaning to exercise more" and then you find yourself saying, "I run" or even, "I am a runner." In a way, the habit becomes part of your identity.

If you have tasted this kind of success before, take a moment to think about how you pulled it off. Was there something about the new activity that you thoroughly enjoyed? Did you find a way to make it super easy? Did you start small? Were you methodical? So often, attempts at creating new habits fail. So, take a moment to consider *why* it worked for you. Write your observations in the space below.

_____

_____

_____

_____

_____

_____

The Palmer Code [Francis Palmer MD]

When you feel you have a clear understanding of why it worked for you before, consider how you can apply the same strategy to the new habits in this chapter that you'd like to establish. Write down three new habits that you think will have the greatest impact on *your number* within the *Palmer Code*.

Habit 1: _____

Habit 2: _____

Habit 3: _____

Now describe how, using your previous successful habit-forming strategy, you might incorporate those habits into your daily routine:

Habit 1: _____

_____

_____

Habit 2: _____

_____

_____

Habit 3: _____

_____

_____

[Francis Palmer MD] **The Palmer Code**

If you haven't had success at developing habits before, now is a good time to start. Perhaps you've wanted to create a good habit but were never quite able to incorporate it into your routine. Perhaps, the good habits seemed a result of circumstance—many of us go through upheavals when we experience trauma such as divorce or a job change and those changes can often result in new life routines. Whatever the case, now is the time to develop the skill of creating good habits. You might want to start small, however and focus on just one good habit to incorporate into your daily routine. To do this, use the same *Palmer Code* strategy you've been following since you started reading this book:

1. Define key elements
2. Evaluate
3. Focus on what's important

Define key elements. During this stage, you simply determine which new habit is going to have the biggest impact on your life and *your number*. Write down that one single habit here:

_____

Evaluate. Take a look at what you're doing now, if anything, that incorporates that habit into your life. Consider ways that you might make it easier, more enjoyable and more satisfying.

For example, suppose you chose "exercise" when you were defining key elements. In the evaluation stage, you note that what you really want to do is compete in a triathlon, but as of now the only exercise you get is a weekly walk with a friend—and you get winded at that! Right now, the point is to make a small, incremental change. You know that walking is enjoyable to you, so perhaps you can talk your friend into going two or three times a week with you instead of only once. If the friend's not up to it, maybe you want to bring along an MP3 player and listen to music or your favorite audio books to keep you going. You might even decide

149

The Palmer Code [Francis Palmer MD]

to set out your shoes and work-out clothes the night before, both as a reminder and to make it easier to get going when the time is right.

Jot down everything you've discovered in your evaluation that will make your new habit easier, more enjoyable and more satisfying:

Focus on what's important. This means you in action as you go forward. This is what's going to help you over the rough patches. Perhaps you've increased your walking and are now bike riding as well and you're feeling fit and fine. Then, something happens to upset your routine: maybe you've been coming home late from work, or you've been sick, or something else happens to cause your fitness level to dip. Remember what's important is the habit itself, not necessarily your level of fitness. If you can squeeze in a twenty minute walk even though you're used to going for forty-five minutes, it's important that you go through the motions anyway, if only to uphold the habit.

A good way to focus on what's important when you're establishing a habit is to use positive affirmations. Perhaps you tell yourself "I am a triathlete in training," even if you've got a long way to go toward that goal. Write down your positive affirmation that will help you keep a daily focus on what's important with your new habit:

Establishing positive habits is one of the most powerful tools imaginable, not only for unlocking *your number*, but also for approaching the rest of your life with a sense of empowerment, confidence and control. You are in control of *your number* and your life. Congratulations for taking the first steps.

Your Palmer Code Self

There are many changes that you can make now, immediately, that can have a drastic impact on your appearance. Some changes may take longer. I encourage you to stick with it and stay true to yourself.

Life and circumstances change, so be ready for anything and try to stay flexible. Maintain your good looks at an early age by using the tips presented in this book. It's so much easier to stay youthful and attractive if you follow small maintenance steps, as opposed to doing nothing until you're 50 and then all of a sudden want to look 30 again. Why not look good as long as you can? Start working early, on improving and maintaining *your number*. Then as you age and find yourself faced with new challenges, you can stay focused and adjust your strategy as needed using the *Palmer Code* to help you pinpoint the areas of maximum benefit. *Your number* is uniquely yours and is with you for your entire life. It deserves your full devoted attention.

Using the secrets contained within the *Palmer Code*, you've fortified yourself with the knowledge you need to reveal your best self and increase *your number*. Going forward, I wish you a long and happy life in which you always look and feel your very best.

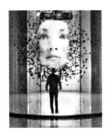

Chapter 15: Afterword

By reading this book you've learned the importance of *your number* and how the *Palmer Code* principles can help you improve and maintain that *number*. From the style of your hair to the food you eat and the strength of your relationships, there are many ways that you can learn to live an enriched and fulfilling life. Yes, the *Palmer Code* shows you how you can be more attractive but I hope that you learned much more. Asking yourself, *"what's my number"* is a question that can be used as a mental exercise; one that encourages you to constantly seek out new ways to improve all aspects of your everyday life. Remember, there's little benefit in knowing that *your number* is an 82. The real power, the real control is in knowing the various ways that you can become an 86, 88, 92 or higher. Perhaps for the first time in your life, you understand the secrets of your beauty, your hidden potential (inside and out) and have armed yourself with the knowledge to create effective and long lasting change not only in your appearance but in all aspects of your life. What could be more powerful and rewarding than your ultimate self-development and improvement?

> "Power, wealth, fame, and charisma are trump cards."

I'd like to briefly touch on the subject of special and unusual circumstances that have the ability to catapult *your number* by 10, 20 points or more. I know you're wondering what these characteristics or traits might be, but once you see them you'll instantly understand

The Palmer Code [Francis Palmer MD]

their significance. *Power, wealth, fame* and *charisma* are the super-qualities that I like to call trump cards because they can have a huge impact on *your number* and how you are perceived by others. We all recognize these traits, and those that are fortunate enough to possess them. Presidents (John Kennedy, Roanld Reagan, Bill Clinton, Barrack Obama), Henry Kissinger, Donald Trump, Brad Pitt, Marilyn Monroe, James Dean, John Kennedy Junior, Princess Diana, Aristotle Onasis and others that I'm sure you can name. These individuals have the ability to captivate our attention. There's little doubt that having one of these super-qualities can transform your life, but they are very rare. If you have one of these traits in the rough, develop it to its full potential as the possible rewards are truly staggering.

I want to leave you with this final thought. Throughout this book, I have shown you non-invasive and non-surgical ways to improve your mind and body in order to make yourself more attractive inside and out. I truly believe that you should try all the easy and non-surgical methods of self-development and improvement first and to their full potential. However, I am a Beverly Hills plastic and cosmetic surgeon that has transformed many lives with aesthetic surgery. I know the transformative power that these procedures can bring. If you've exhausted all the non-surgical options and you are still seeking further improvement in your appearance, plastic surgery may be an option. At that point, I encourage you to learn about the available procedures using the aesthetic principles and guidance you've learned in this book. There are many reliable sources of information on the Internet but here are a few to get you started in your quest.

- My plastic surgery website: http://www.drpalmer.com
- The American Academy of Facial Plastic and Reconstructive Surgery: http://www.aafprs.org
- The American Academy of Cosmetic Surgery: http://www.cosmeticsurgery.org
- The American Society of Plastic Surgeons: http://www.plasticsurgery.org

[Francis Palmer MD] The Palmer Code

Look for my others titles in the *What's Your Number -The Palmer Code* series that will be available in the coming months:

- *"What's Your Number"® Secrets of "The Palmer Code Diet"*

- *"What's Your Number"® "The Palmer Code Exercise Guide for Everyone"*

Get the latest information, book release dates or e-mail your photos for your own *"What's Your Number"®* evaluation at:

http://www.WhatsYourNumberNews.com

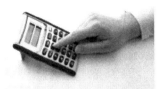

Appendix A: What's Your Number® Worksheet

Use the following worksheet to calculate *your number*. You may want to make photocopies of the blank pages before you fill them out, so that you can have it for future use. Looking at yourself, match your features against the set of examples provided and record the corresponding point value. If you feel that you fall somewhere between 2 examples, decide which one you most closely resemble and take the point difference between the two. For example, if your cheeks look like the example of 70 point cheeks, mark 70 points for your cheek *number*. If you feel that your cheeks are between the examples provided of 70 and 65 point cheeks, decide which one most closely represents your cheeks. Say, it's the 70 point example. If your cheeks are very close to those, your cheek *number* would be 69. If not that close, it's a 68 and so on. Using these simple maneuvers, you will be able to pinpoint *your number* from the set of examples provide throughout this book.

What's Your Number®?

The *Palmer Code* defines the following algorithms and formulas:

Outer you (60%) + Inner You (40%) = Your Number (100%)

Physical Features (80%) + Grooming (10%) + Style (10%) = Outer You (100%)

The Palmer Code [Francis Palmer MD]

Face (50%) + Body (30%) + Skin (10%) +
Hair (10%) = Physical Features (100%)

Physical Well-Being (50%) +
Emotional Well-Being (50%) = *Inner You* (100%)

Use these formulas and fill in the missing blanks to calculate *your number. Let's start with the "outer you".*

Outer you = Physical Features (80%) +
Grooming (10%) + Style (10%)

We can break Physical Appearance down further:

Physical Appearance = Face (50%) +
Body (30%) + Skin (10%) + Hair (10%)

[Francis Palmer MD]   **The Palmer Code**

So let's begin here by calculating these components:

What's Your Number® Face: _____

Cheeks: _____

Eyebrows/Eyes: _____

Lips: _____

Nose: _____

Skin: _____

Chin/Neck/Jaw: _____

Overall Flow: _____

*Total: _____   Fill in Your Face Number above.

❖   ❖   ❖

What's Your Number® Male Body: _____

Torso/Leg Ratio: _____

Shoulders: _____

Chest: _____

Abdomen: _____

Arms: _____

Buttocks: _____

Waist/Hips: _____

Legs: _____

Skin: _____

*Total: _____   Fill in Your Body Number above.

The Palmer Code   [Francis Palmer MD]

What's Your Number® Female Body: _____

Torso/Leg Ratio: _____

Hips/Legs: _____

Breasts: _____

Buttocks: _____

Abdomen/Waist: _____

Shoulder/Arms: _____

Skin: _____

*Total: _____ Fill in Your Body Number above.

❖   ❖   ❖

What's Your Physical Appearance
Number®: _____

Face Number X .50 = _____

Body Number X .30 = _____

Hair Number X .10 = _____

Skin Number X .10 = _____

*Total: _____ Place this number in the space above.

[Francis Palmer MD] **The Palmer Code**

What's Your *Outer you* Number®: _____

Physical Appearance Number X .80 = _____

Style Number X .10 = _____

Grooming Number X .10 = _____

*Total: _____ Fill in *Outer You* Number above.

❖   ❖   ❖

Now, lets calculate y*our "Inner You" Number.*

Inner You = Physical Well-Being (50%)
+ Emotional Well-Being (50%)

What's Your *Inner You* Number®: _____

Physical Well-Being Number X .50 = _____

Emotional Well-Being Number X .50 = _____

*Total: _____ Fill in *Outer You* Number above.

What's Your Number® = *Outer you* X .60 +
Inner You X .40 = _____

Appendix B: Ideal Weight Charts

The best way to determine whether you are overweight is to get a body fat test, either by your physician or through a credible fitness program. A body fat test can be done in any number of ways, though using electronic impulses or a caliber are the most common. As an alternative, you can use the ideal weight chart (table B-1), on the following page, to determine whether you're within your healthy weight range. If you're over or under the range by 15% or more, your health may be at risk and you should talk to your physician.

For women, the ideal weight range is calculated by height and frame size. For men, the range is based on a combination of height and age.

| The Palmer Code | [Francis Palmer MD] |

IDEAL WEIGHT CHART

WOMEN			
Height	**Small**	**Medium**	**Large**
4' 10"	102-111 lbs	109-121 lbs	118-131 lbs
4' 11"	103-113 lbs	111-123 lbs	120-134 lbs
5'	104-115 lbs	113-126 lbs	122-137 lbs
5' 1"	106-118 lbs	115-129 lbs	125-140 lbs
5' 2"	108-121 lbs	116-132 lbs	128-143 lbs
5' 3"	111-124 lbs	121-135 lbs	131-147 lbs
5' 4"	114-127 lbs	124-138 lbs	134-151 lbs
5' 5"	117-130 lbs	127-141 lbs	137-155 lbs
5' 6"	120-133 lbs	130-144 lbs	140-159 lbs
5' 7"	123-136 lbs	133-147 lbs	143-163 lbs
5' 8"	126-139 lbs	136-150 lbs	146-167 lbs
5' 9"	129-142 lbs	139-153 lbs	149-170 lbs
5' 10"	132-145 lbs	142-156 lbs	152-173 lbs
5' 11"	135-148 lbs	145-159 lbs	155-176 lbs
6'	138-151 lbs	148-162 lbs	158-179 lbs
6' 1"	141-154 lbs	151-164 lbs	161-189 lbs
6' 2"	144-157 lbs	154-167 lbs	164-177 lbs
6' 3"	148-161 lbs	158-171 lbs	168-181 lbs

[Francis Palmer MD] The Palmer Code

IDEAL WEIGHT CHART

Height	MEN	
	Age 19-35	Age 36+
4' 10"		
4' 11"		
5'	97-128 lbs	108-138 lbs
5' 1"	101-132 lbs	111-143 lbs
5' 2"	104-137 lbs	115-148 lbs
5' 3"	107-141 lbs	119-152 lbs
5' 4"	111-146 lbs	122-157 lbs
5' 5"	147-150 lbs	126-162 lbs
5' 6"	118-155 lbs	130-137 lbs
5' 7"	121-160 lbs	134-172 lbs
5' 8"	125-164 lbs	138-178 lbs
5' 9"	129-169 lbs	142-183 lbs
5' 10"	132-174 lbs	146-188 lbs
5' 11"	136-179 lbs	151-194 lbs
6'	140-184 lbs	155-199 lbs
6' 1"	144-189 lbs	159-205 lbs
6' 2"	148-195 lbs	164-210 lbs
6' 3"	152-200 lbs	168-216 lbs
6' 4"	156-205 lbs	173-222 lbs
6' 5"	160-211 lbs	177-228 lbs
6' 6"	164-216 lbs	182-234 lbs

Table B-1 was generated from data based on generally accepted systems such as the standard Body Mass Index calculation endorsed by the CDC.

About the Author

Francis R. Palmer III, MD, FACS, creator of **The Palmer Beauty Principles** ™, **What's Your Number** ®and **The Celebrity Lift** ™, is one of the most sought after plastic and cosmetic surgeons in the world.

As **Director of Facial Plastic Surgery for the University of Southern California School of Medicine** for over a decade, celebrities and world leaders alike trust him to improve and rejuvenate their appearance through his unique knowledge of cutting-edge techniques and state-of-the-art technology.

His work is known both internationally and nation-wide as he teaches and lectures about his aesthetic vision and plastic surgery techniques. Dr. Palmer frequently appears as an expert on plastic surgery in both scholarly and general media and serves as a consultant for emerging technologies in the aesthetic industry.

His recent accomplishments include creating **The Celebrity Lift** ™, which takes substantially less time to perform and less healing time than a conventional facelift. He is known for **The Palmer Beauty Principles** ™, his system of beauty principles and his **"What's Your Number"** concept that guide his acclaimed aesthetic work on people from all over the world.

A Pennsylvania native, Dr. Palmer has called Southern California home for over thirty years. An honors graduate of San Diego State University, he received his MD from the University of California – Irvine.

Following his residency at USC-LA County Medical Center, Dr. Palmer completed a fellowship with the American Academy of Facial Plastic and Reconstructive Surgery and is board certified in that specialty. He has also completed a fellowship with the American Academy of Cosmetic Surgery and is board eligible in that specialty.

Dr. Palmer and his expert plastic surgery techniques have been featured in many broadcast and print media, including ABC's The View, CNN, ABC, CBS, NBC and Fox News, Dr. Phil, Entertainment Tonight, Allure, Fit, USA Today, Cosmopolitan, US Weekly, People, In Touch, The New York and Los Angeles Times. British magazine *Tatler* named him "one of the world's best plastic surgeons." Even renowned columnist Liz Smith has mentioned Dr. Palmer.

Dr. Palmer has created his own line of cosmeceuticals, **Francis R. Beverly Hills**, that produce for book younger looking, healthy skin that radiates wellbeing.

When Dr. Palmer is not in surgery or devising a new procedure, he loves to paint in acrylics, watercolors and oils. Many of his canvases hang in his Beverly Hills office. He resides in Santa Monica with his wife and two children.

http://www.drpalmer.com   http://www.whatsyournumbernews.com

Book Bonus

As a special offer, *What's Your Number*® will be offering three audio recordings that you can find on the web site by typing in the url **http://www.whatsyournumberbook.com/bookbonus**

The three audio recordings will be added material on *"healthy eating-because diets don't work"*, *"exercise by the numbers for the body shape you really want"* and *"commonsense numbers approach to your life and relationships"*.

These three topics are setting up our subsequent book releases in the *What's Your Number*® series that will be

1. healthy eating/diet book
2. exercise book
3. positive attitude/relationship building book

Dr Francis Palmer

BUY A SHARE OF THE FUTURE IN YOUR COMMUNITY

These certificates make great holiday, graduation and birthday gifts that can be personalized with the recipient's name. The cost of one S.H.A.R.E. or one square foot is $54.17. The personalized certificate is suitable for framing and will state the number of shares purchased and the amount of each share, as well as the recipient's name. The home that you participate in "building" will last for many years and will continue to grow in value.

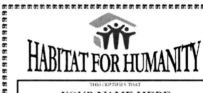

Here is a sample SHARE certificate:

YES, I WOULD LIKE TO HELP!

I support the work that Habitat for Humanity does and I want to be part of the excitement! As a donor, I will receive periodic updates on your construction activities but, more importantly, I know my gift will help a family in our community realize the dream of homeownership. **I would like to SHARE in your efforts against substandard housing in my community!** *(Please print below)*

PLEASE SEND ME _____ SHARES at $54.17 EACH = $ $_____

In Honor Of: _____

Occasion: (Circle One)   HOLIDAY   BIRTHDAY   ANNIVERSARY

   OTHER: _____

Address of Recipient: _____

Gift From: _____   *Donor Address:* _____

Donor Email: _____

I AM ENCLOSING A CHECK FOR $ $_____ PAYABLE TO HABITAT FOR HUMANITY <u>OR</u> PLEASE CHARGE MY VISA OR MASTERCARD *(CIRCLE ONE)*

Card Number _____ Expiration Date: _____

Name as it appears on Credit Card _____ Charge Amount $ _____

Signature _____

Billing Address _____

Telephone # Day _____ Eve _____

PLEASE NOTE: Your contribution is tax-deductible to the fullest extent allowed by law.
Habitat for Humanity • P.O. Box 1443 • Newport News, VA 23601 • 757-596-5553
www.HelpHabitatforHumanity.org

Printed in the United States
153981LV00013B/75/P

の講義をしっかり学べば読解力も鑑賞力もじゅうぶん身につくはずである。にもかかわらず、そこにあえて「文芸翻訳演習」という科目を加えたのは、「訳読」を先鋭化して「翻訳」という明確な目的を提示するためである。さらに、学生たちは翻訳という作業に憧れにも似た感情を有していることから、「自分は今この授業で翻訳をしているのだ」という充足感も与えることができる。

さて、その「文芸翻訳演習」の授業をどのように展開するか。わずか15回の授業で、将来の翻訳家養成を目標とすることはできない。また、斎藤兆史氏が2007年に『翻訳の作法』で示しているような水準の授業を本学で行うことも難しい。受講生はある程度の語学力はあるものの文学的教養は拙い学生たちである。しかし、その一方で彼らは「勤勉さ」という翻訳という作業にとって何物にも代えがたい長所を備えている。以下は、そのような学生を対象とした「文芸翻訳演習」の2014年度と2015年度の実践例である。

7.4　2014年度の実践

「翻訳研究II」という科目名称であったが、文芸翻訳の授業は2014年度にスタートした。受講生は英語英文学科の2年生から4年生の12名であった。全員英検2級以上の英語力がある。授業では、英語読解上重要でありながらも学生がつまずきやすい項目を択び、①例題を用いた説明、②短い文の翻訳練習、③30語から60語程度の課題演習（2題出題することもあった）、という流れで進めた。③については授業の2日前の正午までに訳文を担当者にメールで送るよう指示し、担当者はそれを添削し、次の授業の冒頭で簡単なコメントとともに返却し、さらに陥りやすい誤りや優れた訳については書画カメラ（OHC）を使って紹介・説明するようにした。

各回の授業の項目と狙いは以下のとおりである。

第1回：人称代名詞
〈狙い〉he, she をいつでも「彼」「彼女」と訳していては日本語にならない。逆にこれをうまく処理すると日本語らしい表現になる。このことに加

7.3 積極的訳読主義としての「文芸翻訳」

　語学力の向上のために文学作品を読むのは、その言語のもっとも優れた表現が文学作品にあるからである。筆者自身そう教えられ、今もそれを信じている。コミュニケーションの道具として英語を駆使することの重要性、あるいは楽しさは微塵も否定する気持ちはないが、そのコミュニケーションにしても文学作品を知ることでさらに豊かになるはずである。また、映画などのサブカルチャーも文学作品を土台にしていることが多いため、それを知っていれば理解もさらに深まり、会話も盛りあがるはずである。

　本学に限らず、現在、英語英文学科に入学してくる学生の多くは英語でのコミュニケーション能力を身に付けることに最も大きな関心がある。新入生に日本文学、外国文学を問わず何か文学作品を読んだことがあるかと尋ねても、高校の教科書以上の回答は得られない。もちろん、シェイクスピアもディケンズも読んだことはない。しかし、内容的には稚拙ながらも、先に紹介したような1年次の読解の授業を通して、あるいは入学後の何かを契機にして、文学作品を読むことの大切さ、おもしろさに気づく学生も確実に存在している。そして、そのような学生の多くは一定以上の英語力を有す勤勉な学生であり、「文芸翻訳演習」は彼らの文学的、語学的興味の受け皿として成立する。

　文献や作品を正確に読むために、「訳読」型授業は必須である。もう30年近く前になるが、ケンブリッジ大学での在外研修の機会を与えられた。当大学を選んだのは筆者が研究している E.M. フォースターの母校であり、著名な研究者もいたためだが、1年間の研修中に日本語学科の教員たちに会う機会を得た。そこで、日本語能力の向上のためには何が必要かと尋ねたところ、即座に translation だとの答えがあった。彼らと「外国語を読んで適切な母語に置き換えることのできない場合は理解がじゅうぶんではない」という考え方を共有できたことは、イギリス小説の研究者であるとともに語学教師である筆者にとってその後の大きな支えとなった。

　訳読型授業は、本学のカリキュラムでも Reading や日本人の担当するゼミナール（複数履修可）などいくつか並んでおり、これらの授業とともに専門